Advance Praise for *Get Lost*

"Erin Leider-Pariser takes us on an expeditionary sojourn of body, heart, and soul. We discover that pilgrimage, when led with care, strengthens the body, opens the heart, and ultimately liberates the soul. The lessons she shares are jewels of life's path."
—**Lisa Miller**, Ph.D., bestselling author of *The Awakened Brain: The New Science of Spirituality and Our Quest for an Inspired Life*

"This wise, funny, and honest book brings new meaning to the spirit of adventure. Erin Leider-Pariser shows us how to leave our comfort zones for journeys that challenge the body and feed the soul—all while having a roaring good time. *Get Lost* dares us to engage with the world and each other in new ways to find the meaning and happiness waiting for us around the next curve of the trail."
—**Dan Buettner**, National Geographic Fellow and #1 *New York Times* Bestselling author of *The Blue Zones*

"I knew Erin-Leider Pariser was a kindred spirit when she told me her adventure trips always have a philanthropic purpose that supports the places she visits. Agreeing on such things, including my motto that "Everything is possible—the impossible just takes more time!" made my decision to guide Erin's group in Nepal an easy one. My wish is that this wonderful book will stimulate people to see more of the natural world, because awareness is the first step in solving the challenges our planet faces. Read, enjoy, and get out there!"
—**Johan Ernst Nilson**, explorer, philanthropist, and award-winning adventure activist

"I went on many of Erin's adventures with small groups of women, trips that were arduous, challenging, breathtaking, and filled with so much laughter my belly hurt. There was love and beauty all around. At the end of each one, our hearts were filled with goodness, kindness, and gratitude. We could then go out into the world and spread the joy."

—**Cheryl Tiegs**, entrepreneur, actress, and former supermodel

GET

Lose Yourself to Find Yourself

LOST

Seven Principles for Trekking Life with Grace
and Other Life Lessons from Kick-Ass Women's Adventure Travel

ERIN LEIDER-PARISER

Post Hill
PRESS

A POST HILL PRESS BOOK
ISBN: 979-8-88845-074-1
ISBN (eBook): 979-8-88845-075-8

Get Lost:
Seven Principles for Trekking Life with Grace and Other Life Lessons from
Kick-Ass Women's Adventure Travel

Cover design by Jim Villaflores
Cover photograph by Susan Barron

Excerpt from In-Q, "Say Yes, Inquire Within." Used with permission of the author.

Excerpt from Margaret Noodin, "A Joyful Life," as published in Heid E. Erdrich, Ed., *New Poets of Native Nations*, Graywolf Press, 2018. Used with permission of the author.

Talking stick photographs by Susan Barron

Post Hill Press
New York • Nashville
posthillpress.com

Published in the United States of America
1 2 3 4 5 6 7 8 9 10

To all my inspiring teachers and mentors,
the family I was born into,
and the family of friends and adventurers I created,
all of whom have made me who I am.

TABLE OF CONTENTS

Go some place you've never gone.
Some place that will scare you some.
Be someone you've never been.
You feel all that adrenaline?
It's medicine to jumpstart the spark inside your skeleton.
See? Everywhere you are is where you're supposed to be.
So hopefully, you're hopelessly
as lost as me.
'Cause if you're not, you ought to be.

— "Say Yes, Inquire Within" by *In-Q*

INTRODUCTION

We use the word *friend* so casually that we forget its
power and depth.... The love and understanding
of a friend, like a deep well of the purest water,
refreshes the very source of our being.... As we bring
our vulnerability, insight and heart into conscious
relationship, we realize we are all waking up together.

—TARA BRACH[1]

ON A MISTY NOVEMBER MORNING in the pastureland of Ecuador,
a local shaman led me and my small group of women adventure
travelers toward an array of giant ceremonial pyramids from the
thirteenth century. After burning a stash of herbs and snorting
tobacco, he began his spirit cleansing ceremony by placing his
hand on my head to pull out any negative energy and, with a
push-and-pull motion in the air above, replace it with positive
energy. Grimacing with intent one moment and widening his
eyes with charged energy the next, he seemed to transform into a
different person before our eyes. We stood among the sacred pyramids for hours as he performed the healing ceremony on each
of us individually. At the end of the afternoon, feeling incredibly
peaceful, we made our way back toward the hacienda.

All the trips I have arranged for women through my company, Sports Travel Adventure Therapy (STAT), over nearly three
decades have offered a spiritual element of some kind such as the
shamanic healing we experienced in Ecuador. Thanks to STAT, I

---

1   Tara Brach, *Radical Acceptance: Embracing Your Life With the Heart of a Buddha*,
    Random House, 2004, pp. 297–298.

have found a way to live my purpose: to inspire women to leave their comfort zones and find missing pieces of their lives through journeys into the wilderness and the soul. In these pages I share our stories of personal growth, physical renewal, and spiritual discovery to reveal how bonding and friendship can transform women's lives.

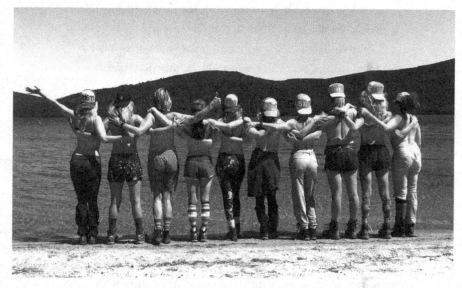

Baring our souls in Tasmania. *(Photo: Author's Archive)*

At the center of this book are insights I have gleaned from our travels about how to live life to the fullest, a set of guidelines that can help us *trek life with grace*. My Seven Principles for Trekking Life with Grace are: 1) Nix the Competition; 2) Walk with Integrity; 3) No Judgment; 4) Start with Effort, Finish by Grace; 5) Mark Your Words; 6) Love, Honor, and Obey Your Intuition; and 7) Embrace Community. In early 2020, my habit of (usually) following the sixth principle about intuition led to writing this book. What seemed like just a minor skiing accident turned out to be a nudge into taking on a challenge I had never dreamed of—if I was willing to listen. As I always say, there are no accidents, no coincidences…only synchronicities.

On that bright, snow-glinting day in Aspen in the first week of January 2020, I had just come home from taking my favorite King yoga class, and I felt amazing. As usual, this therapeutic style of yoga left me feeling deeply relaxed thanks to gently loosening my ligaments and bringing my bones and muscles into what felt like perfect alignment. I poured a glass of green juice and sat at the kitchen counter, relishing my contented state of mind and body. My husband Paul breezed in and suggested we spend the gorgeous morning hitting the slopes for a quick ski down Roch Run. My first reaction—the silent, intuitive message from my gut—was, *no way, not when I'm so relaxed and loose; the last thing I should do right now is ski down a bump run like Roch.* But Paul was so cheerful and the sunshine so dazzling that I ignored that little voice in my head.

Once we were on the chairlift up to Roch, the little voice kept pestering me, but who hasn't hushed up their intuition from time to time? That's always a bad idea, as this day would once again remind me. Sure enough, on my first run, my ski caught an edge and I went down. I felt okay, so I got up, brushed myself off, put my skis back on, and kept going. Paul and I met up at the end of the run and took the chairlift up for another go. *Uh-oh.* I told Paul I needed to go in because something wasn't right. Going "in" meant stopping at the restaurant just a few yards away, a popular spot on top of the mountain. We sat down for lunch and I pulled off my boots. By the time we finished, my right knee had swollen up and sprouted splotches of purple. I couldn't put on my right boot, so Paul helped me limp out to the gondola for a ride down the mountain to town. The scenery was spectacular, but little of that registered because all my senses were preoccupied with my throbbing, eggplant colored knee.

It wasn't that bad, I told myself, in denial that I could hurt myself on a slope I'd skied many times, so I asked Paul to take me to my physical therapist instead of the hospital. The PT put some electric stimulation around the knee for the trauma and told me to go home and ice it. When I woke up the next morning, my knee had blown up—it was huge. We went to the emergency room and the x-ray showed I had fractured my tibial plateau, the upper part of the shin bone that settles into the knee. The doctor wrapped it up and sent me home with instructions to put no weight on the leg for at least two weeks.

What a calamity. I thrive on routine and ritual, and with my entire active-and-fitness-oriented lifestyle disrupted I lost my grip. When people called to ask how I was doing I would break down in tears. My immobility hit me like a truck, leaving me disoriented and sad. I had to find something productive to do, so I told myself, when you can't be out there, you have to get *in* there. I had to regroup, pivot, and get introspective.

My first impulse was to recap what I was grateful for, and my STAT community was high on the list. As the "no coincidences" universe would have it, I had already decided to take a break that year and not schedule any trips. There I was, no planning to attend to and all the time in the world to reflect on the past twenty-eight-plus years of life-changing adventures with curious, wise, courageous, and wild and crazy women. Little did I know a pandemic that would shut down the world was just weeks away, which, combined with my free time and storehouse of experiences, would create the perfect setup for writing. I'll never forget the moment I saw the opportunity for writing this book spread out before me with every piece magically in place. Even if I had planned on a new year of STAT trips, COVID-19 would have canceled all of them, so my earlier decision to take a year off seemed downright prescient. My skiing accident threw me out of my normal life and demanded I get reflective, turning my bed-ridden situation into fertile ground for dreaming up this book. My only question was, if I had listened to my intuition and not skied that day, would I still have this book in hand? I believe my spirit, the universe, God, or whatever you choose to call it would have found another way to inspire me to write about these unique experiences.

Through two years of COVID I gathered together lessons learned and used my field notes to share details about some of the challenges we've put ourselves through and places we've explored around the world. (None of the women who have joined STAT trips are professional athletes—our physical prowess runs the gamut from daily walker to yoga teacher and hardcore runner—and our trips accommodate all these levels.) I highlight the inner/outer adventure stories of women like Shannon, who decided to follow through with our trip to Tasmania after being diagnosed with breast cancer. The entire trip was a lesson for Shannon in letting go of control and learning to be calm in the face of new terrain and physical challenges. Back home, her new centeredness made all the difference during her weeks of chemotherapy. I tell the life-changing story of Susan, who was so moved by the needs of the children she met during a trip to Phnom Penh, Cambodia, that she wrote up a business plan for a charitable organization on the flight home and ran that program full time for the next decade, outfitting thousands of children around the world with school supplies and later serving military families.

Before delving into those stories of transformation and lessons learned, I share the beginnings of my journey from a cheerleader kid in Miami to one of the first trainees in the Jane Fonda fitness method in Los Angeles. My evolution from a personal trainer to the stars in New York to trekking the world with women to help them grow into their best selves is followed by an exploration of my Seven Principles for Trekking Life with Grace.

In the final pages I reflect on life lessons from the COVID era and offer a roadmap for setting up your own adventure travel circle with your friends. My greatest wish is that this book will light a spark in you to form that travel group and kick off a new level of connection and personal discovery with your "tribe." Any nature-steeped destination will do, from a nature park near home to one of our national parks to a land across the sea. What matters is your willingness to exercise your body, mind, and spirit as a group with a common sense of adventure and trust.

Strengthening our friendships brings many remarkable, scientifically proven benefits to our health, wellbeing, and sense of connection to our fellow humans across the world, as I review in Chapter 10. As media scholar Douglas Rushkoff writes, "Being human is a team sport.... Anything that brings us together fosters our humanity."[2] These advantages, however, almost pale alongside the sheer joy of being together in the great outdoors to rediscover our authentic selves. On hikes along Spain's ancient Camino de Santiago trail, walks across rice paddies in Cambodia, rugged climbs in the Canadian Rockies and past waterfalls in New Zealand, and mountaineering hikes up the moss-covered Kii slopes of Japan, we've put our bodies, minds, and spirits in motion to learn from nature and each other. How could I keep all this collective wisdom to myself? How could I tuck in a notebook the firsthand knowledge that our friendships—with all their caring, laughter, and hilarity—are literally our lifelines? Hospice chaplain Kerry Egan, author of *On Living*, reminds us that our friendships are vital to our ability to live our purpose:

> We live our lives in our families: the families we are born into, the families we create, the families we make through the people we choose as friends. This is where we create

---

2   Douglas Rushkoff, *Team Human*, Norton, 2019, p. 3.

our lives, this is where we find meaning, and this is where our purpose becomes clear.[3]

This book is a love letter to all the women who have journeyed with me and every woman exploring life beyond the everyday. My decades of adventure travel, near and far, convince me that taking part in a travel circle of your own will kindle a new dimension of friendship courtesy of Mother Nature and your courage to explore the unknown. I hope this book will inspire you to ignite that adventurous spirit and take bold new steps toward your dreams.

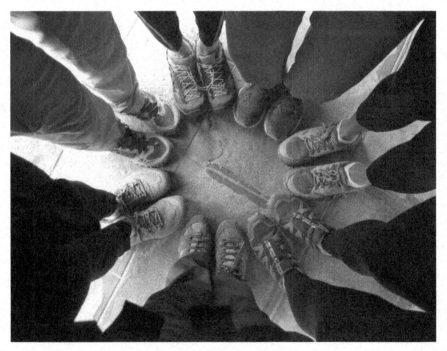

(Photo: Judy B. Nussenblatt)

3   Kerry Egan, *On Living,* Penguin, 2016, p. 28.

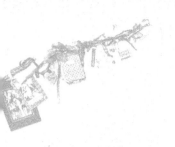
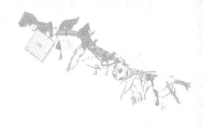

PART I

PASSION
AND PURPOSE

Who we are matters immeasurably more
than what we know or who we want to be.

—Brené Brown[1]

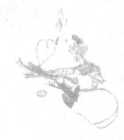

1   Brené Brown, *Daring Greatly*, Avery, 2012, p. 77.

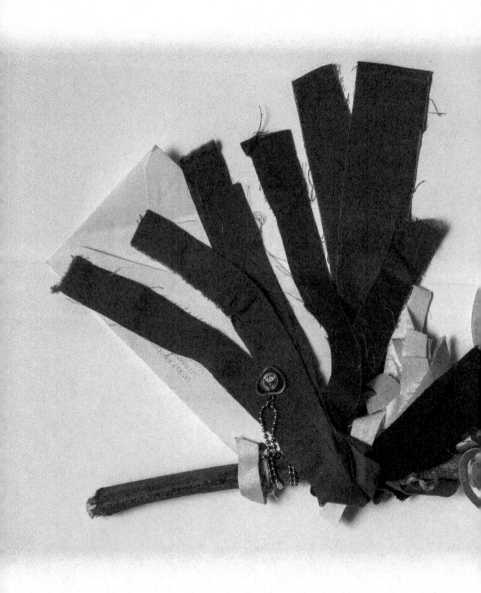

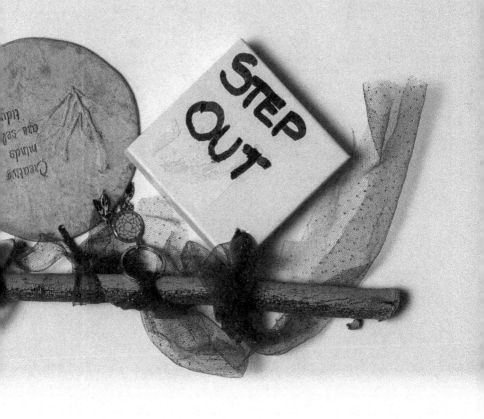

CHAPTER 1

"EXERCISE WITH ERIN"

Give with love. Give in joy. More you cannot do. Less
you must not do, if it is your intention to be of service.

—IYANLA VANZANT[2]

MY CAREER FOUND ME.

That's how I feel about life—life finds you. There are no accidents. The universe gives you clues along the way, and you have
to be open to them. It's like a treasure hunt, and you can't miss
one of those clues. If your mind is open and you're quiet enough
to listen, life finds you. That's why I meditate and hike with only
my pups (first with Sydney and now with Sadye), to hear what
the universe has to tell me, because you can't really hear from the
inside when you're busy with everything else.

The other night I listened to an interview with Delilah, the
radio host whose call-in show came out nationally in the 1990s.
Hearing her voice brought back memories of listening to her at
night as callers shared their personal stories of love and loss. She
was a natural at giving advice and matching up an experience
with the perfect song. In the interview, she talked about the early
days when she was trying to launch her show. Producers kept
telling her it wouldn't work, that people wouldn't respond to it.

2   Iyanla Vanzant, "November 1," *Until Today! Daily Devotions for Spiritual Growth
    and Peace of Mind.* Atria/Simon & Schuster, 2000.

She got hired and then fired for talking too much, but she never gave up. Now she's a radio icon.

Delilah's story reminded me of the obstacles that came at me when I was deciding whether I should start a women's adventure travel business. A lot of doubts, excuses, and reasons why it wouldn't work shouted me down…but they were all in my head. It would take an adventure of my own to hear my truth and make that decision.

Now, as I look back and follow the thread that weaves through the past sixty-four years, I see that I was getting ready for my career—I almost hate to call it that, because it's so much more—from the beginning. As a kid, I loved sports. It went with the territory, because even though I was the third of three girls, I grew up as the son my father never had.

MIAMI BEACH

It's easy to play outside a lot in Florida, because we only have one season. There are dry months and wet months, and that's it. So I was physically active all the time, and by the time I came along my dad was semiretired, so he had a lot of time for me. He sold his insurance company when he was relatively young and parlayed that check into a lot of little businesses that kept him not too busy and very happy. He had been in the right place at the right time with that sale, and I may have gotten the best part of the deal.

Most of my quality time with my dad was spent on the driving range, but he also took me to a lot of games. I was in the third grade when the Miami Dolphins started up, and we went to all their games. Sitting in the stands with dad, the hot dog guy stopping by in his paper hat, the announcers' voice bouncing off the far fence…it didn't get any better than that. Since my sisters were six and eight years older, in some ways I was an only child and treated like one. I became the boy in the family, playing football, softball, and soccer on the street with the boys and a few other girls and heading to all those games with my dad.

There were no girls' sports teams in those days, so cheerleading was a big deal if you were athletic. I was a cheerleader in middle school and then became the captain of the squad at Miami Beach High School. We practiced like crazy and I was the short one who always jumped to the top of the human triangle and did the splits. I tried to date the quarterback—so typical—and my friend Marjorie, whose dad played golf and poker with my dad, was a cheerleader with me all those years. We also went to summer camp together, along with another friend, Alison, and they are both close friends to this day who have been on many of my Sports Travel Adventure Therapy (STAT) trips. It's funny how Marjorie still talks about how badly she feels about earning the White Pine Award at camp one year while I didn't win anything. It didn't bother me to not be recognized for my leadership and all-around good camper status at the time, and still doesn't, but that's a friend for you. On one of our trips, Marjorie and Alison gave me an honorary Red Pine award, gifting me a pinecone with such sincere intention that it felt like receiving an honorary degree from Harvard!

My dad was a happy-go-lucky man in every sense of the word—with three daughters he couldn't have been happier, and he was lucky in life. Mom and Dad wanted us to get an education and be happy, healthy, and do whatever we loved. Mom found and lived for her purpose, which was us. She was a war baby, a woman from a generation whose goal was to get married and have children and do the best she could with raising those children. She insisted on her daughters getting an education, and her greatest aspiration was to see us build happy lives. That's the story of many women from her generation. My dad died young and my mom did the best she could with the tools she had.

Neither of my parents pressured me to get a job or career and strike out on my own as soon as I graduated from college. I think there are two ways to look at that: If somebody lights a fire under your ass, you do what you have to do. If I had developed a little more ambition to make more money, maybe I would have. But if you're not given that kind of ultimatum as you start out, you're more on your own to be driven by things that become important to you. That's how it worked for me, and I'm grateful for it.

The travel bug bit me hard in college when I took a semester abroad in London. I met my friend Susan when we were both attending Boston University, and that semester we covered so much ground we felt like real Europeans. I planned trips, meticulously, every weekend. We went to Edinburgh. We went to Paris. I got us Eurail passes and we visited Israel and Greece, including the Greek Islands. It was so easy to jump on a hydrofoil or train and be in another country in an hour. I stole time in the evenings to pore over maps on the little desk in our dorm room and figure out where we should go next and what we must see while we're there. I loved working out the details, and only later would I realize that the smooth sailing and joy of the trips we packed into those weeks were a hint of things to come.

I had chosen to study public relations/communications at Boston University, but I didn't know what I would do with it. I wanted to be in a liberal arts program and didn't really think about what I was going to do for the rest of my life. Writing, communication, and journalism classes sounded like an interesting starting point. I was learning how to observe and pay attention and then describe what I saw. There was a difference between watching and really seeing something, and as I explored Boston, seeing started to feel like a show of affection. To *see* the tree standing between the sidewalk and the Chinatown Arch was to feel all that life as it contrasted with the concrete and brick, and I connected with it in a powerful way. The tree was a stranger like the people rushing around me, but a calm one, and a force that held so much energy it had to press itself out in tapering leaves. How could you not love such a thing?

Boston was really cold for a Miami girl, though.

After my second year I headed back south and transferred to the University of Florida at Gainesville and graduated from there with the same degree.

JANE FONDA LAND

With no pressure from the folks, I struck out on my own after college, moving to L.A. to take a job writing articles for a small publication in an insurance company. I settled into an apartment with a childhood friend, Mary, who was living near UCLA in Westwood and needed a roommate—great timing. After my nine-to-five job every day I'd go to a gym to run and work out, but I soon learned about an exercise class in Beverly Hills that was taking the city by storm. This was 1980, and Jane Fonda had recently opened a studio on Robertson Boulevard called "Jane Fonda's Workout."

On my first visit the place was packed. Instructors led workouts in three connected studios that surrounded a patio space, and within a half hour I was in one of them with about forty other men and women in shorts and cropped t-shirts or high-cut leotards and tights. As we stretched, twisted, and lunged, we'd glance out at the patio, hopeful for a Jane sighting.

That night I got my first dose of the music-backed aerobics that would launch a national fitness craze and change the country forever. The moves were fun, the music got your blood pumping, and the crowd vibe was a blast. No wonder three thousand people were coming through the door every week. Jane, who had for years done ballet for exercise, wore ballet leg warmers in her workouts and set another trend that swept the country. *Jane Fonda's Workout Book* came out the following year and was a number one *New York Times* bestseller for two years. Next came her two-album *Jane Fonda's Workout Record*, which I still have, and then, in 1982, the world's first fitness video, *Jane Fonda's Original Workout*.

In the two years I went to class and trained at the Workout, I never saw Jane, but I loved the social aspect of it. I didn't get hired to run a class, either, but I must have made a good impression because I was invited to be in the cast of the Workout play. Yes, they tried to do a stage play based on the Workout—so Hollywood! I played one of the people in the class, just like I had been doing three nights a week after work, and we rehearsed at the studio every night for about eight months. We didn't get paid, but it was an honor to be asked to be in it. Exercise was in my DNA, and I guess it showed because they only chose the best students who were training at the studio. I don't know what happened, but the project never got off the ground and the whole thing fizzled out. It was fun while it lasted, but for Jane's Workout, the play was not the thing.

Jane's training program was taught by one trainer who had been taught by Jane herself. After two years in that program I knew the Workout inside out and was full of ideas for how to make it my own. The fitness craze was in full swing and it seemed like a great time to get back to the East Coast, so I planned a move to New York. I enjoyed my writing job and the Workout, but for the most part Los Angeles was a hard city for me. I didn't have many friends there and everything was so spread out you had to drive everywhere. It was time to move on.

Fitness mania had definitely hit New York when I returned in 1982. At the center of it all was the new Vertical Club on East 61st Street, one of the first workout studios in the city. After getting certified as a fitness instructor through the Athletics and Fitness Association of America (AFAA), I applied at the Vertical Club and was hired to teach classes using my own method.

The Vertical Club was big. Not just in popularity—I mean big as in huge. No one had seen anything like it. You walked into this giant industrial space with a running track lining the perimeter up above and windows offering a stunning view of the Queensboro Bridge. The factory-size floor included a stage on one end for instructors to lead aerobics classes that held a hundred people at a time. Weight machines and other equipment shared one section of the floor, leaving plenty of room for the classes.

The energy in that place was fantastic, and members really responded to my playlists that accompanied each part of the workout. It didn't take long for them to memorize the moves as they came back multiple days each week. Some of those songs still ring in my head, like Survivor's "Eye of the Tiger" that I used for an ab routine and Peter Allen's "Quiet Please, There's a Lady on Stage" for our cool down at the end of the workout.

I was known for my key songs and took pride in how I curated my music. My classes became very popular at the Vertical Club because I tried to make it entertaining for everybody. It felt more like fun than work, just a bunch of people motivated and upbeat and inspired by the moves, the music, and each other.

All eyes were on me as I dictated orders, and little did I know in those first months that one guy doing his laps on the running track was checking me out too. Paul Pariser, a handsome New York native working in commercial real estate, eventually signed up for my classes. As it turned out, we had a mutual friend, my childhood pal and fellow cheerleader Marjorie, who had also moved to New York. She introduced us. No coincidences, right? Paul and I started dating and kept seeing each other after I left the Vertical Club in 1984.

Since my workouts were getting so much attention I decided to break out on my own at the end of that year and rent a studio to run my own classes. My new business, "Exercise with Erin," offered classes as well as private, one-on-one sessions. Things really took off as word spread, and three days a week at 5:30 p.m. people crammed into my walk-up studio at the Douglas Wassell School of Ballet and Theater Dance located in the Ed Sullivan Theater on Broadway. We got hot and steamy in that studio with my boom box blaring to George Michael singing "I gotta have faith, faith, faith" and Glen Frey belting out "The heat is on!" In the summer I spent the weekends in the Hamptons running classes in a studio that a woman named Gala had opened up at the Bridgehampton Surf and Racquet Club. She called her exercise studio "Galasthenics." Writers, actors, and actresses escaping the city flocked to those sessions, and after leading a couple of classes I could spend the afternoons at Bridgehampton Beach.

For all the fun I had, I looked at my new venture as serious business. Some of the weekend warriors around the country were getting hurt putting their bodies through high-intensity work-outs and yoga sessions that their bodies weren't ready to do. I wanted to delve deep to learn more about the body and how it works, so I decided to enroll in the two-year Exercise Physiology master's program at Columbia University. In the mornings I sat in beautiful, theater-like lecture halls with big windows and learned about muscles and movement, anatomy, nutrition, how to do research, and a lot more. It was such an honor to be in those classrooms. The rest of the day I met with clients, ran my studio workouts, and had a lively social life with my friends. In the midst of this crazy, exciting time, Paul and I got married.

We took our vows in May 1985 at the Water Club on the East River, where the view of the Manhattan skyline to the north and south is spectacular. My family flew up from Florida and Paul's came from his hometown on Long Island, and of course many of our friends were there. As you can imagine, it was a big hair, big sleeves, totally 1980s affair.

The next year, when I was brainstorming about what to do for my research project in the MA program, I got pregnant. I decided to do my paper on pregnancy and exercise, studying how the body shifts in terms of the bones and ligaments and undergoes other changes. Part of my research involved field work talking to gynecologists about what pregnant women should and shouldn't do. Those doctors were very conservative back then. They encouraged their patients not to do anything because they were nervous about any kind of exercise. This was before we had any studies on these things. Are you supposed to stop running when you're pregnant? Yes, the docs said. Today the answer is no—you should basically continue everything you've been doing because your body has a memory and adapts to the changes that come with the pregnancy. You shouldn't start something new, but it's safe to keep up a lot of your regular exercise and activity. Based on my studies I transitioned into doing a pregnancy exercise class for a while. I wasn't the only one—many exercise studios began offering classes for pregnant women in New York

City at that time. It became a new norm that continues today, and gynecology has had to evolve along with it.

SWEATING WITH CHERYL

My new credentials helped me get more clients and word started to spread about me among the celebrity crowd. Everyone had fitness mania, and the prospect of having a pro come into your home at your convenience was a huge draw. I visited one of my first celebrity clients, supermodel Cheryl Tiegs, three times a week in her beautiful apartment on Park Avenue. Before I came along, Cheryl got most of her exercise doing a ton of walking around the city. I would show up, pull on my leg warmers, click "play" on my boom box, and we'd get to work. She always made time for laughs and chit chat, especially when she learned that Ivana Trump was one of my clients. She was always asking things like, "What kind of nail polish does Ivana wear?"

The funny thing was, Ivana always asked me about Cheryl too. "What does Cheryl do for a workout?" "What does she wear?" "How does she work the waist?" I never talked about my clients, but I could tell she wanted to be friends with Cheryl. Ivana was a very regular client because she had been an athlete most of her life and loved to work out. Growing up in Czechoslovakia, she learned to ski at age four and was a competitive skier before moving to Canada, where she worked as a ski instructor and model before coming to the United States. I spent quite a bit of time with her, showing up at the Trump's apartment in Trump Tower around 8:30 or 9:00 in the morning three days a week for at least five years (Donald always answered the door). Ivana had a special room just for exercising, and she was delightful—so warm, friendly, and respectful. She may have been part of New York's social elite, but she had no qualms about dripping sweat all over her designer workout wear and marble floors in order to stay in great shape.

All of my clients found me through word of mouth—I never had to advertise "Exercise with Erin." I doubt the one-page promotional piece with logo (shown below) I typed up ever made it into anyone's hands because the clients just kept coming. Part of my little promo read:

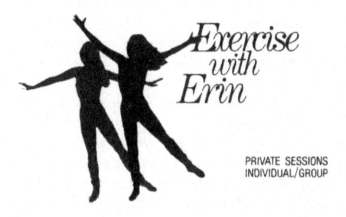

Exercise with Erin

PRIVATE SESSIONS
INDIVIDUAL/GROUP

Being a forerunner in the spread of private and personalized workouts, she created her own business called "Exercise with Erin." She provides the opportunity for people with children at home, working people, people interested in anonymity, and people with special physical limitations the plain luxury of being energized on an individual basis in your own home.

What sets Erin apart is her genuine affection and understanding of each of her clients. She adapts her workout to her clients changing schedules, physical abilities, moods and lifestyles. She believes in working hard and playing hard, with exercise as the equalizing agent. Most of all, exercising with Erin is fun. She is a perfect wake-up call, a mid-morning break, an afternoon Snickers bar, or an evening wind down.

My high-profile clients worked in many glitzy sectors. Someone in the TV industry who lived in my building introduced me to Barbara Walters, who, unlike Cheryl and Ivana, hated to work out. She had a sensitive back, so we concentrated on strengthening her abdomen to give her back more support. We would set up in her foyer, the biggest open space in her Park Avenue apartment, and I'd help her exercise with a pair of little hand weights. Many of my clients were couples, like artist James DeWoody and his then-wife Beth who is an art collector and philanthropist, and Alan Gottlieb and his wife Ann who was famous for her professional "nose" in the designer fragrance industry. Paola Schulhof and her friend Penny Glazier were regular clients, and they introduced me to another famous couple in their building, songwriter Neil Sedaka and his wife Leba. The first workout with the Sedakas those mornings was moving furniture to make room, but thank God the grand piano could stay put.

My celebrity clients needed me to make them exercise. They had a lot of other things to do, and after we got to know each other some just wanted to visit with me and not do the work. We became good friends because we spent a very intimate hour together. They talked about their lives and confided in me, and I just listened. When they were going through challenges and feeling vulnerable, I think they liked having someone to talk to who wasn't judgmental or in their circle of well-known friends. Sometimes I'd come in and they'd say, "Let's just have coffee" or "Have you had breakfast?" It was very tempting, but I never gave in to them. "No," I'd say, "let's go; we'll just do a little," and I'd get them started. There were days I'd get to Cheryl's place and she'd say, "I'm feeling so down today," so I'd tell her to put her sneakers on and we'd go for a walk in the park or walk up and down her building's stairs a few times. Stair climbers were getting very popular in the 1990s, but as I told Cheryl the first time I led her to her twenty-story stairwell, "Who needs a Stairmaster?" Cheryl and I walked a lot of stairs together.

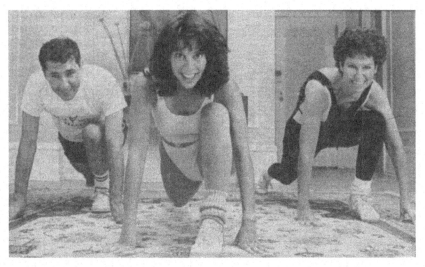

Working out with Alan and Ann Gottlieb in their home, from an article about personal fitness that appeared in the *New York Post* on September 23, 1986. *(Photo: Author's Archive)*

Working with all kinds of New Yorkers on their fitness and wellness was deeply gratifying as well as a lot of fun. I felt I was being of service in a meaningful way, which is the secret to happiness. Our network of friends kept growing, and when we weren't having dinner parties we'd meet at our favorite coffee shops and restaurants. Living in a city I loved, surrounded by friends and our growing family of two small boys, my heart was full. But change was in the air. In 1995, my work and social life dissolved like sugar in a cappuccino.

As our boys were reaching school age, Paul wanted to move out of the city. We talked about it, and I had to agree that it may be better to raise them in a place with more room to grow and play. Our sons were four and seven when we moved to Greenwich, Connecticut, about thirty-five miles north of Manhattan. It was just an hour's drive from the city, but a world away as far as I was concerned.

I started to trek into the city at least three times a week to meet clients, but the commute and hassle became too much. It just didn't work for me. Firmly settled in Greenwich, I needed to be more than a carpool mom, but I didn't know how I was going to find anything that could replace the high-energy, rewarding career I had worked years to build up. At least I knew that finding a new goal would mean listening for clues from inside and out. As writer Iyanla Vanzant puts it, "Your spirit cannot show you the way until you are clear about the direction you want to travel."[3]

I didn't need to be anxious, just patient. The intuitive nudges I soon felt and followed proved that my spirit had a plan to not only show me my direction, but also how to get there.

---

3   Iyanla Vanzant, "January 3," *Until Today! Daily Devotions for Spiritual Growth and Peace of Mind.* Atria/Simon & Schuster, 2000.

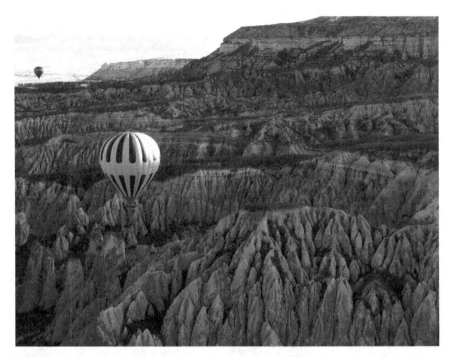

Letting the wind determine our direction over Cappadocia,
Turkey in 2011. *(Photo: Judy B. Nussenblatt)*

CR

FOR REFLECTION

1. Are any of your childhood friends still in your life? How often do you talk or meet?

2. What was your first act of independence as a young adult?

3. If you were a teenager or adult in the early 1980s, did you get into the fitness craze? (Do you still have your Jane Fonda album?) If you started exercising at that time, did you enjoy it enough to keep up an exercise routine to this day? Or, if Jane Fonda's fitness mania was before your time, do you exercise to online videos by today's fitness gurus or at a club?

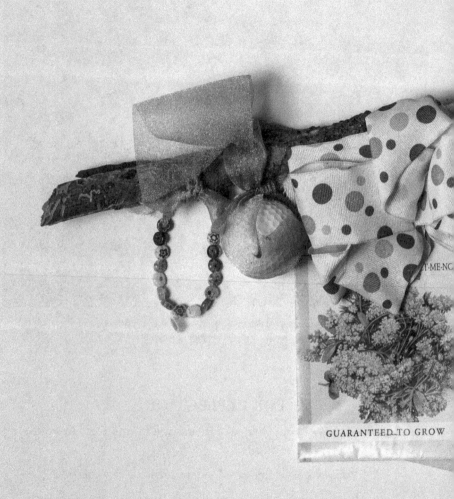

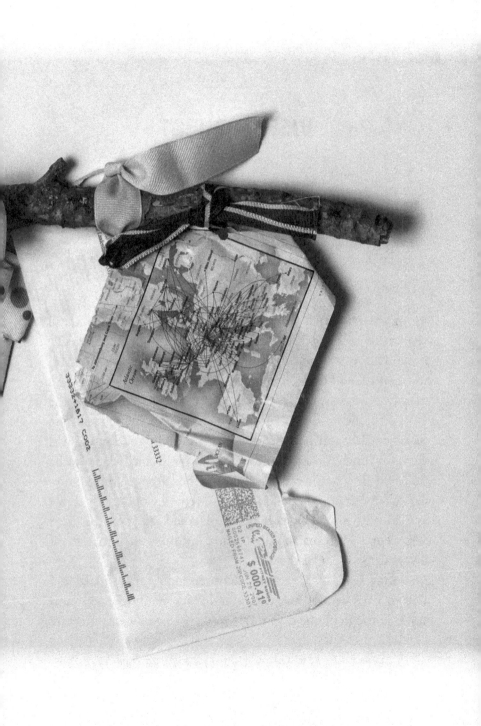

CHAPTER 2

VISION QUEST

In our lives, even though one episode amounts
to a crash and burn, there is always another
episode awaiting us and then another.

—Clarissa Pinkola Estés[1]

After phasing out my commutes to New York City, I still
saw one regular client who came up to Greenwich on weekends.
Ivana Trump wanted to continue exercising with me, and in
addition to working out in her Greenwich house, one weekend
she invited me on the family's private plane to Mar-a-Lago, the
Trump's home in Florida (as if you didn't know). I taught exercise
classes for her and her friends in the morning and then joined
them for lunch, outings, and dinner. Ivana seemed elated to be
surrounded by her eclectic groups of friends, from European royalty to famous fashion designers, who were all wonderfully down
to earth and embracing. My husband would say I was the hired
help when with Ivana and her friends, but I never felt that way. I
always felt like one of the girls.

Seeing Ivana in Greenwich kept reminding me of the fun I
used to have with all my clients and made me miss them even
more. Through phone calls and letters, I learned I wasn't the only

---

1   Clarissa Pinkola Estés, *Women Who Run With the Wolves*, Ballantine, 1995, p. 220.

one. Many of my regular clients wanted to get together for exercise and camaraderie, and the fresh Connecticut air must have been getting to me because I decided to organize a trip and take Exercise with Erin on the road. I planned for six of us to meet up in Wyoming to trek in the Grand Tetons for a group vacation with me as the fitness guide.

As I made the calls and received the Exum Mountain Guide Brochure, I was intrigued by the description and photos of the climbs. I talked one of my friends into joining me for the trip with its potentially challenging climbs because this friend was always ready for adventure—a real trooper. We once climbed an indoor wall in Vail, Colorado, together and absolutely loved it. Wasn't that enough experience to climb the Grand Tetons? Not quite. Most people go to the basic climbing school for two days before becoming eligible to climb them. We didn't have two days to spare in our upcoming schedule in Jackson Hole, Wyoming, however, so we spent one day in New Paltz, New York (two hours from New York City), with an accredited climbing instructor. Two of the women who would join us in Wyoming attended the training, too, but decided that climbing wasn't for them.

After numerous conversations with our recommended climbing instructor, Jim, and trekking guide, Becky, we organized an itinerary so my friend and I could climb the "Grand" and still meet up with our four friends the next day to trek as planned.

She let me do all the planning while she did all the worrying. She asked a few times about the trip and I answered vaguely, concerned that she wouldn't climb with me if I told her too much. I intentionally avoided getting all the details on the climb myself. The brochure said that no prior experience was necessary to climb the Grand. That's all I needed to know. Even Jim said, "Everyone does it." Most of all, I wanted my friend to climb with me because that would legitimize it. This woman is a thought-out, disciplined person, while I am impulsive. Besides, doing this climb alone, given my lack of experience, would have been questionable.

The first day of the climb was a strenuous 5.5-hour, 8.5-mile hike up to the lower saddle base camp. Elevation 11,002. The non-technical climb brought us across lots of huge boulders traversing with one freestanding rope up a ravine. My partner was strong and impressive. We got to the hut, essentially an oversized tent that sleeps sixteen very tightly, in time for our boil-in-a-bag dinner and a brief talk about the actual climb and equipment.

Jim told us about our 3:00 a.m. wake-up. Everyone must begin their actual ascent up the Grand no later than 4:00 a.m. to avoid the storms up top that roll in every day at noon. The night was very windy, sixty miles per hour. We didn't sleep at all.

We started our climb in the dark with no flashlights, just the light from the stars. It was pretty incredible; Jim had it down to a science. I had no idea what lay ahead for us, but I trusted him and kept thinking of his comment that *everybody* does this climb. I probably took that quote out of context, but I love challenges. My friend was scared. She said on more than one occasion that she wouldn't go. Jim thought that she just wanted to be coaxed, so he played up to her by saying, "Oh come on, you can do it!"

We were fully clothed in our long underwear, pile pants, pile jacket, wind pants, wind jacket, wool hats and gloves, harnesses, ropes, carabiners, figure eights, chalk bags, and helmets. It was cold and windy in the dark—awfully creepy, but exciting.

But my fellow climber was not happy at all. We took it slowly. As we got higher, the exposure got greater. She was expressionless, on the verge of tears. Five-and-a-half hours into the climb, most of it non-technical rock hiking, we were on the easiest route called Owen Spalding. However, we were totally exposed, looking thirteen thousand feet down, if we dared to look at all. We were in the middle of nowhere, if you call the Grand Tetons nowhere.

Rock climbing is a mental game, and once you get spooked it's hard to recover up there. Jim pulled me aside to tell me that my friend was not going to make it. She was petrified, totally frozen at the limbs, and we still had seven hundred feet of technical climbing left to the summit. After he showed her the rest of the climb from where we were, she turned to me and said, "Erin, I'm sorry, I can't do it." At that moment, I felt my excitement drain and my chest tighten up. I wanted to reach the summit so badly and I knew that the only reason she had come this far was not to disappoint me.

We had four days of trekking with our friends ahead of us, and I was concerned that her anxiety would turn to anger towards me, if it hadn't already. I remembered many times when my anxiety turned to anger for not being able to handle a challenge. I then realized that my friend was scared, not angry. She wasn't being selfish, just thinking about my disappointment.

The entire way down, I tried to work it out. I became introverted. The disappointment was overwhelming. I had this unfulfilled feeling. I kept thinking about the climb, trying to figure out how I could have finished while she went down or waited. I reached the same conclusion each time: we were in it together or not at all. Why was it so hard to leave it at that? It must be that only-child syndrome, even though I'm not one, or that type "A" competitive, controlling personality. After all, this was a pleasure trip, and besides, the Tetons weren't going anywhere. We had the rest of the week to enjoy stress-free trekking in this magnificent landscape with a couple of friends and the pals they brought along. The day after our climb attempt, my fellow adventurer and I met up with them and the rest of the week was sheer joy. Six female city slickers in the mountains of Wyoming, taking it all in.

My unfinished climb in the first days of that trip taught me a lot about myself. I realized that I had approached the whole thing with an obsession to summit, to complete what I started, to focus on the end result no matter what. Thanks to my friend's disruption of that, I was able to reflect and develop a new perspective about climbing and everything else: it's not about the summit or goal—it's about the journey. It's about being in the moment with all its sights, smells, sounds, textures, fear, love, curiosity, and beauty. We have to enjoy the journey while we can. A few years later another mountaineering trip confirmed my new view.

To celebrate my fortieth birthday, Paul and I set off for Mount Kilimanjaro in Tanzania, just across the southern border of Kenya in East Africa. Kili isn't the tallest peak in the world, but at 19,551 feet it is the highest freestanding mountain on Earth and the tallest mountain in Africa (by comparison, Everest is 29,029 feet and Alaska's McKinley is 20,322 feet). The aerial view on Google Earth showed tropical forests covering about two thirds of the mountain on all sides until giving way to meadows, desert uplands, and snow-covered rock. As we discovered, the ascent through those misty forests is steep. You get into high altitudes quickly. As we neared nineteen thousand feet I began dry heaving every ten minutes. Altitude sickness is common on Kili, regardless of how fit you are. I had made it near the final summit, but I knew I couldn't go any further. I turned to Paul and said, "I gotta go down."

"Thank God you said it," he told me. "That makes me the happiest person in the world." He didn't want me to push myself beyond my limits and get sicker, but he didn't want to tell me to stop, either. The old Erin, before my first Grand Tetons climb with my friend, would have kept trying to lurch along to reach the top between hunching over with stomach spasms. But the forty-year-old Erin was fine with turning around when her body said no more. Just setting foot on Tanzania, seeing with my own eyes why Kili is called the "roof of Africa," and trekking up a good part of the mountain was one of the biggest thrills of my life.

SEDONA

The women's Wyoming trip turned out to be more than a vacation with friends. The positive group vibe inspired me to plan another trip, this time taking a bigger group to the Southwest. That second trip would become a bridge between the career I was leaving behind and the new chapter life had in store for me.

By the mid-1990s, Sedona, Arizona, had become ground zero for the New Age. I had read about its vortexes, centers of intense, spiraling energy that draw people who claim these centers can recharge and heal. The photos I'd seen of the valley town, which has been called one of the most beautiful places in the country, also made it irresistible. Red rock formations and buttes surrounding the valley, giant saguaro cacti, white and purple phlox spreading across desert rocks…no wonder so many Westerns were filmed there. I made plans for our group of twelve to camp out under the stars and experience some rugged hiking and whatever Sedona's fabled spiritual mix had to offer.

My old friends Alison and Marjorie were game for the adventure, as was Cheryl, who by this time had a baby. We were all in our thirties with young children, and at the time Marjorie was feeling that she had somewhat lost her voice, her sense of self. One day, when one of our hikes turned into a rigorous climb, she seemed to find it again. "On one part of the hike we had to go up this sheer wall with finger holes," she recalled, continuing:

There was a moment when, my face against the rock, I was between the group who had made it all the way up and the girls below, and I heard one after the other tell me, 'Move your right hand here,' and 'Move your left leg there,' until I finally got to the top. *Yes, I did it!* I thought. Some people look before they leap, and then don't leap, and some people just leap. I'm a more cautious person, but climbing up that rock face was the beginning of proving to myself that I could do anything.

Cheryl faced down her fears on that same challenging hike along the Cathedral Rock Trail. She says my sense of humor was the only thing that got her through parts of it, but I knew how strong she was, inside and out. "There was a time I had to spider walk, two hands, two feet, against rock that was grainy from the weather," she said. "I looked over my shoulder and thought, if I start sliding, that's a thousand feet down, and there's no going back with only those little crevices in the cliff." Once she made it to the small, flat tabletop, she saw herself reflected in another climber's eyes:

As we sat up there, they started handing out sandwiches. I have a fear of heights and couldn't look over the cliff because it was right there and it was so windy. I was so scared. I had a two-and-a-half-year-old waiting at home for me and I thought, I've got to get down off this rock. I looked at the girl across from me and she was looking at me and probably thinking the same thing, since she had just had a baby. On the way down the other side with our guide we were able to hold onto a rope and eventually get to a path, but it was very slippery. That downward hike was even scarier than the climb. Marjorie started singing because that's what she does, and because we were all scared and it was so steep, and Erin kept talking and making us laugh because that's what she does. After another half day we made it to our campground and went to sleep on sacred Indian ground. We heard chanting as we closed our eyes.... I guess that was our reward for what we'd done.

I learned an important lesson on that trip that I would take with me when I eventually launched my adventure travel business. Our guides that day had not been up front with me about the rock face climb that lay ahead. If I had known, I would have made the guides describe the challenge beforehand so the girls could decide whether to take that trail or not. Choosing guides carefully and asking questions to be clear about what's in store is critical.

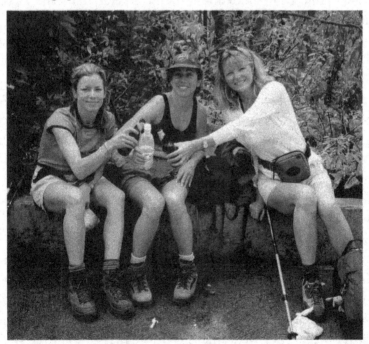

Left to right: Deborah B., Jodi S., and Cheryl Tiegs celebrating our ascent up Machu Picchu. *(Photo: Author's Archive)*

The nighttime chanting Cheryl remembered was a hint of the spiritual essence that filled Sedona. We were told that a massive spiritual vortex covered the entire area in addition to the smaller vortexes mapped out in specific places. One night we took part in a sweat lodge ceremony, letting the heat penetrate our bodies and open our hearts. Based on the Native American ritual, the sweat ceremony was infused with symbols, from the round shape of the small covered lodge that represented wholeness and the womb of the Earth to the prayers that called to the four sacred directions, another connection to wholeness. We crawled inside on our knees, moving clockwise to take our places on the ground.

A man brought in sparkling volcanic stones that glowed orange from being heated in a fire for several hours and placed them in the shallow pit in the center of the space. Then the water pourer entered and closed the flap behind him, leaving us in pitch darkness except for the superheated rocks. He ladled water onto the stones and sat near the flap as thick steam poured over us. I suddenly understood why we had been given a handful of sage— holding it over my nose and mouth protected me from breathing in the worst of the heat. For the next nearly four hours we let the heat melt away our comfort zones, leaving us open to surrender and clarity. We prayed, we sang, we sweated and detoxed inside and out. Between rounds, the water pourer opened the flap and let the cool night air creep in, refreshing us just enough to be ready for another foray into letting go.

Two women in our group, Cristina Carlino and Jennifer Stockman, bonded during the ceremony because they bowed out of the last two rounds together, crawling outside to breathe freely and talk about what they experienced in the altered state of the sweat. They were strangers before that day, but the sweat opened them up to themselves and each other, and three decades later they are still friends. Inside the sweat lodge, I had my own revelation about bonding. Drenched from head to toe in sweat and tears, I felt the power of sitting with women in a sacred place. What would it be like to create opportunities like this for women each season of the year, exploring the world with a focus on nature and spirituality? That was the gift of my first sweat lodge ceremony, a new openness to possibility. At the same time, doubts crept through my open pores. Imposter syndrome kicked in. Who was I to think I could start a travel business? I didn't have any training or professional experience, and my first job was to be mom to my boys. I had no idea in that moment that my new friend Cristina would help steer me away from those doubts and toward a new adventure as an entrepreneur.

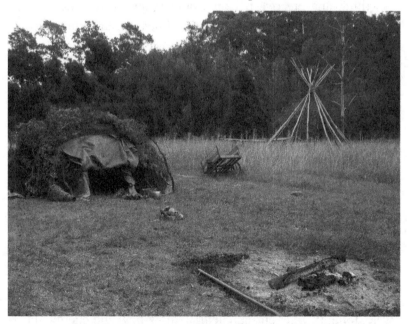

A present-day sweat lodge, or temazcal, in Mexico, with the fire pit in the foreground. We participated in the ritual in a similar temazcal on a trip to San Miguel de Allende. *(Photo: Temascal by Mgodiseo, 2008. Public Domain, https://commons.wikimedia.org/wiki/File:Temascal.JPG)*

At the time, Cristina was beginning to develop her Philosophy skincare line, which would become one of the most popular brands on the market with its messages of inspiration and holistic wellbeing. Her story about how her unique vision for this line came to her is spiritual in its own way. When I heard that story, I wasn't surprised at how much she loved our little group's time together in magical Sedona. As she told me, her business idea appeared to her during her usual morning hike on Phoenix, Arizona's, Squaw Peak (since renamed Piestewa Peak):

I was alone on Christmas morning, a career girl, crying, having a pity party, when suddenly there was this giant rainbow in front of me. In that moment I had what I think any creative person would know of as a 'download,' an input of all the parts and pieces that ultimately became Philosophy. Everything came at one time. That universal download said here's the blueprint, now go do it. I felt I had permission to go do it, so I did.

When she joined us on the Sedona trip, Cristina was working on Philosophy out of her Phoenix office and the brand had not yet launched. Soon after I returned home from those four magical days of hiking and sweating and bonding, she called me and encouraged me to create a business of my own. She had been taking note of how I handled myself, my friends, and every situation that week and thought I was a natural to go professional with the women's trips I loved to arrange. "I see in one second, clear as a bell, what a person can and will do," she recently told me. "It's seeing something in such a simple way, and when I met you, you were doing it." Her entrepreneurial know-how and energy didn't let up—she called me every day that week like a mentor on a mission. Carlina claims I was a pack leader through and through who just needed a "little nudge," but her influence was much bigger than that. She gave me a lot to think about.

COLORADO QUEST

My good friend Jody was always ready to listen when I needed to sort something out. A budding Waldorf teacher, she had recently moved from Connecticut to Boulder, Colorado, seeking Waldorf education for her children. She was looking for an alternative lifestyle and could relate to my need to explore new ideas, so she invited me to come to Boulder to see her. She arranged for us to attend a Zen retreat for three days and then go on a vision quest to dig deeper into finding my purpose. When she told me that the leader of her woman's group (which they affectionately called "the witches") ran a women's vision quest retreat in one-and-a-half-mile-high Estes Park, I was sold.

Jody couldn't have chosen a more perfect way to get into the self-reflective zone than the Zen retreat. We got up at 4:30 each morning for two to three hours of group meditation in a beautiful, wood-and-stone constructed circular room. Toward the end of each session we went into walking meditation around the inner circle. Everyone helped with the cooking, and most of the delicious meals were eaten in silence. In our free hours we hiked some stunning trails. Who knew that gathering together to enjoy scenery, good food, and simple tasks like doing dishes and sweeping up without saying a word to anyone could be so powerful? The non-verbal environment made us pay closer attention to faces and expressions, the taste of the food, the plates and bowls we held, and how we carried ourselves. Everyone's gestures were as peaceful and gentle as the trees, grass, and plants around us. After the third night it was time to drive north for the next adventure, and our conversation had a quiet new feel. We were ready to get up another mountainside to spend a few days with the leader of the witches.

Jody and I showed up at a rustic wooden house in the wilderness outside the town of Estes Park, more than seventy-five hundred feet in altitude with a spectacular view of dozens of peaks in the North Range of the Rocky Mountains. People flocked to the town as a way station for visiting Rocky Mountain National Park and to stroll through the charming shops, but I hadn't come all this way to be a tourist. Our trip led us to a wooded property containing a little house that held four sets of bunk beds and no shower. For the next three days and nights, Claudia McLaren Lainson, who was a leader at the Waldorf School, guided us through a life-changing journey of self-reflection.

Claudia's rituals, borrowed from Native American traditions but tailored as her own, included a talking stick ceremony that began with her bringing a bare, yard-long tree branch to our circle around the campfire. Claudia was a beautiful woman with blue eyes and long gray hair pinned up loosely to leave two long strands framing her face. She looked into our eyes as she explained that the ritual provided a way for each of us to describe our individual essence. Each person holding the stick would speak, without interruption, about who she was at the core, what made her tick.

Earlier in the day we had expressed that essence in an artwork project, selecting items from Claudia's box of arts and crafts supplies to create a little masterpiece that symbolized our true self. The symbols we had chosen for that art piece, including the materials and shape, revealed our individuality in ways that words alone couldn't convey. We went around the circle with the talking stick to describe the layers of meaning in our artwork and how they reflected our deepest selves. Claudia spoke with utter confidence about her inner life and spiritual outlook, things most of us had never tried to share with anyone, creating an atmosphere of reverence as we watched the sparks float up to the sky.

The next evening, after a day of solitary walks along deer trails through the aspen and spruce and long conversations about our dreams and other inner experiences, we made beef and vegetable soup in the tiny kitchen. The pot stayed on the stove while we went back outside to take part in Claudia's version of a sweat lodge ceremony. She made it clear that she was not appropriating this sacred ritual from Native American culture, which would have been disrespectful, but forming a ceremony inspired by that tradition. We bent down to step into a round hut covered in a canvas tarp and blankets with a pit dug into the center. The grass felt cool on my bare legs as I sat cross legged a couple of feet away from the pit. Claudia poured a bowl of cold spring water onto the stones and the hut clouded up in steam. The heat felt more intense than in the sweat ceremony I had experienced a year earlier in Sedona. She told us there would be four rounds to the sweat and we could leave at any time if we couldn't take it.

Instead of praying to our ancestors, as the water carrier in Sedona led us to do, we were led in a series of prayers and chants that Claudia began and we repeated. Claudia's ritual invoked a strong feminine presence that wound through and around us as we let our bodies surrender to the heat. As I closed my eyes and breathed through the fabric of my t-shirt I had pulled over my nose and mouth, images floated through my mind like pages being swept away from the loose binding of a book. In one, I am sitting on a boulder in the Lotus position in the center of a circle of women facing me in the same pose. That image gives way to one in which I'm looking over my shoulder at the woman below me as we climb the gentle slope of a mountain. We're laughing with joy. Next, I'm walking a trail with thick brush on one side and the sea below on the other, carrying extra water canteens strapped across a heavy pack on my back, last in a line of about eight women. The salty air is wet on my face and arms and a woman up ahead sings a cheerful camping song that drifts over the trail. Everyone is happy and full of energy. I'm smiling because I made this happen—I brought them here and they trust me. They know I'm strong enough to have their back.

By now, we were near the end of the third round of the sweat, and as I slipped back to reality the heat hit me hard. I started to panic, knowing there was no way to move my body that would bring me relief. I got on my knees and started for the rug-flap of a door, but Claudia cuts me off. "Please try to hang in there," she said. "You have to sweat it out." I moaned and shook my head. "I can't. I can't breathe and I think I'm going to pass out."

"What's blocking you?" she said as she crouched down next to me. "There's something going on; you have to let it go! Kiss the ground—the air is slightly cooler there. Get your head into the dirt. Get to the core of who you are! Find out why you're here!"

She was such a powerful woman. For a moment I thought her belief in me meant I was safe and could get through it, but then I felt myself slipping away and said, "No, I have to go out. I have to get air—now."

She let me crawl past her and said, "You can go out if you have to, but you'll need to work. You're not leaving the ceremony." She followed me outside and handed me two large sticks. "Use these to pass me the rocks so I can bring them in for the next round. You're going to work through this." The fresh air cleared my head immediately and I shoved the sticks beneath a rock at the top of the glowing pile. I dropped it into the bowl she was holding and quickly turned around to pluck up another. When the bowl was filled enough she took it into the hut and returned to me a few seconds later to start again. I felt my biceps clench as I lifted another rock. The stones nearer the bottom were slightly larger and I squatted to use my legs instead of my back. The work was slower this time and I was sweating again. I was amazed at Claudia's strength as she held that large bowl of stones. After I piled on about the sixth rock, she went back through the opening and shut the makeshift door behind her. "I guess that's it," I said.

I lay down on the spot and let the night air cool me down. We were far enough from town that the darkness brought out the most glorious night sky I'd ever seen. Maybe the altitude made the stars look so bright. I felt tiny in the face of the mountains that drew a jagged line against the starry sky. Words from Onondaga (Iroquois) Chief Oren Lyons in a book I had back home came to mind: *We stand somewhere between the mountain and the ant.* Lying there beneath the universe I felt much closer to the ant.

The clarity of the air, stars, and sky matched the clear vision sweeping up from my heart to my head. I saw that my place was in the center of a yoga circle where women's feet pressed into the ground and the wind played in our hair. My place was at the top of a climb and the back of a trail. It was in the company of women who wanted to connect with nature, their bodies, and themselves. Okay, I told myself, I get it. I can do this. Here in the starlight, grounded on the Earth, I've made my decision.

At the end of the final round of the sweat, Claudia and the others stepped out of the hut and I joined them inside the house for soup. Jody walked around the table dropping cilantro leaves into each of bowl to add fragrance to the beef, potatoes, carrots, onions, celery, and peas that had stewed together over the past three hours. I was empty through and through and the room smelled like heaven.

The next morning, we made coffee over the campfire and Claudia gave us directions for our last solo hikes. I wasn't angry at her for pushing me so hard the night before; on the contrary, I was grateful that she'd taken me to the edge where I could find my truth. She smiled as she guided us on how to walk mindfully to find a place to sit and meditate alone on whatever came up, maybe the intention we set the first night or something revealed during the sweat or in a dream. We would know the place when we found it.

After breakfast, I walked for about fifteen minutes until I came to a stand of aspen trees. After sitting for a while, I lay down to stare up at the delicate flipping leaves. Gratitude flooded my heart. Sunlight blinked between one set of branches and slowly moved up to the next. I dozed off a few minutes at a time, but not deeply enough to stop hearing the woodpecker tapping several yards away. Nothing pressed my mind for answers because I felt as secure in my purpose as I had the night before. I felt light and steady as I imagined where I could take my first travel adventure group. Cristina's voice bubbled up from memory: *I see in one second what a person will do.* I finally saw it too, and I shook my arms and legs with excitement like my boys do in a pile of leaves. I'm going to do it! Yes—I'm going to do it!

I can create this experience for a lot of people on my terms, I told myself. These small-group trips could have a transformational effect, something everyone was looking for at the time. (The times had become ripe for natural foods too—years later Jody used her grandmother's beloved granola recipe to launch Boulder Granola, branding her very successful homespun product with the tag line "Unleash your inner hippie.") The whole country seemed to be obsessed with finding meaning through ancient wisdom, nature, sacred places, meditation and yoga, crystals and channelers. People were asking the big questions: Who am I? Why am I here? What's the point of it all? I could give women a chance to find the answers, one trip at a time. Where should we start? I let that question drift by as I relaxed again beneath the leaves. When the sun glided into the spot directly above, it was time to head back for lunch.

STAT!

As soon as I got home from Colorado, Cristina helped me turn my dream into reality by using her design and marketing staff to draw up and print my first Sports Travel Adventure Therapy flyer. Seeing my business name in print for the first time…priceless. My vision of creating a way for women to find their true selves, to transform and heal through adventures in nature with kindred spirits, was now a real thing.

The four-word name I chose for the business not only described the elements that would go into each trip, but also added up to a stable-feeling square. My venture, STAT, felt grounded, and at the same time the acronym suggested quick, active movement by echoing the medical word for "immediately:" *Get me a scalpel, stat!* Everything felt right.

Cristina gave me access to her business expertise and office equipment whenever I needed it. Her talented people taught me how to design my own flyers, and over the next twenty-plus years I would have a great time writing up highlights of locales and how we would play in them. Over the next year, Cristina launched Philosophy and invited some of us from the Sedona trip to her exclusive events in New York City. We were both off and running, me with women's travel adventures—and my own printer!—and she with her skincare line. Our paths did not cross much after that, but Cristina was instrumental in sprouting my wings for my new life, and I will always be grateful to her for it.

My simple yet official-looking first STAT flyer went out to my friends and former clients who shared it with their friends, and within a couple of weeks I had whittled down a sizeable group of interested travelers to eight. I wanted to keep the groups small. Our maiden voyage, a whitewater rafting trip on Idaho's Salmon River, would take us to the West that attracted so many seekers at the time. I felt like we were part of a grand trek to places steeped in legends of energy vortexes, supernatural ley lines, and geo-spiritual doorways that could unlock the secrets of life and the universe.

Or maybe we were just in for some awesome scenery.

⌘

FOR REFLECTION

1. Did you explore any New Age practices in the 1970s or 1980s, or if you're younger, do you read about or participate in any similar activities (Eastern philosophies, yoga, spirituality, etc.)?

2. Has a friend or mentor motivated you to make an important decision or take a certain path? If yes, do they know they've had this positive influence in your life?

3. Have *you* helped a friend or family member make a big decision about their life?

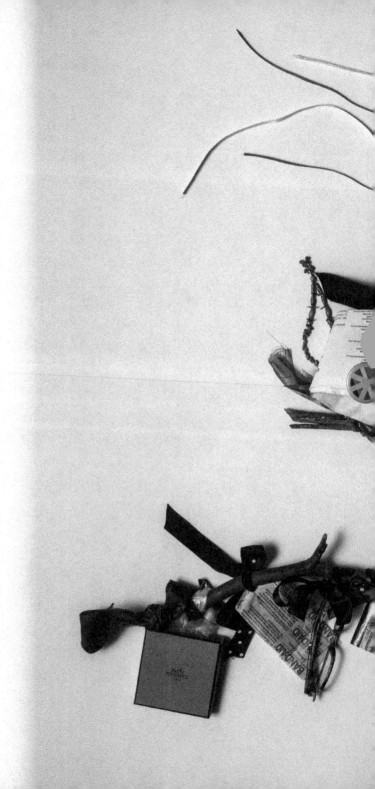

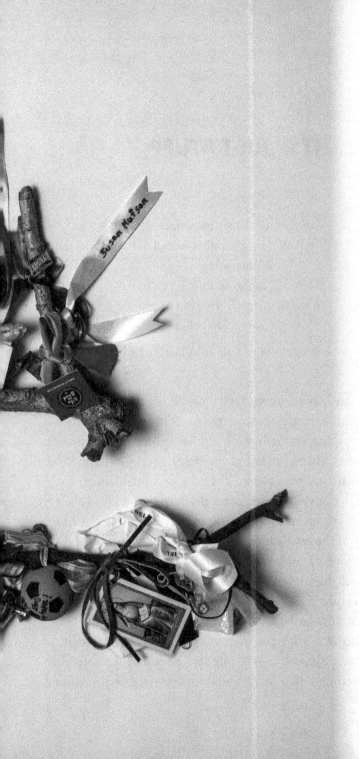

CHAPTER 3

IT'S JUST STUFF

It's easy to change our minds
to look through a window, fall
into a lake
it's harder to quit,
to wait or step off the main path
to discover a joyful life.

—Margaret Noodin, from "A Joyful Life"

THE SILVER THREAD RUNNING THROUGH all my travels, from the
earliest onward, is made of two strands. With each adventure I
discover something about myself and something that connects
us to each other, thanks to the group experience. Over time I've
discovered that this two-layered thread also runs through each
friendship, relationship, and activity that graces my life. When I
pay attention, a conversation in line waiting for coffee can be as
enlightening as the revelations that await on a wilderness trail or
within a ceremonial circle.

A personal insight that would develop into a staple of each
travel agenda popped up as I prepared for the first "official"
Sports Travel Adventure Therapy trip to Idaho's Salmon River.
That early autumn I learned that my intuition is more than a
reliable source of guidance—it can also be a creative force for
birthing something original. I wanted to offer the group a talking

stick ceremony like Claudia had provided in Colorado, but I needed to make it my own. Like Claudia, I respected the sacred Native American origins of the ceremony and did not want to appropriate a piece of that culture, so I followed my hunches to dream up a different take on the tradition. While Claudia had focused on the ceremonial talking stick circle as a gateway to our inner selves, my intuitive imagining led me to envision the experience as a way to define and express a specific intention. Sitting together, each woman could describe something they wanted to manifest in their lives. To get the most out of the experience, I decided to ask them to bring something from home that represented their intention and would be attached to the talking stick when it was their turn to speak. This would allow them to give their manifestation the attention it deserved while preparing for the trip. Inspired by Claudia's method of asking women to craft a symbol of their deepest selves, I zeroed in on a practical purpose for a ceremony that could provide a safe space for sharing personal insights we rarely get to talk about with anyone else.

In a note or call to everyone about a month before that first trip, I described the talking stick ceremony and asked them to start thinking about the intention they would like to share and the item that would symbolize it. I waited until the final four weeks before the trip to reach out about this because I wanted them to think about something current. They would not get their symbolic item back, I said. Instead, it would become part of a collection that would forever be part of the group. The idea was generally well received with a few hesitations and questions like—*What if my insight is something I don't want to tell anyone about? What if I can't think of anything I really want to manifest?* I encouraged them to be as deep or shallow as they like—no pressure, reminding them that everyone would be in the same boat (or raft) and that the point of the whole trip was to step out of their comfort zones a bit. No one would force them to say anything. I told them to just go with it and an idea would inevitably come up and they'd be fine.

I slated the talking stick ritual for the second night of the Salmon River trip. Day one would give us time to get to know each other as we rafted with our onboard guides several miles down the middle fork of the Salmon River, easily navigating rapids that were tamer that time of year. For five hours we floated in dumbstruck awe down clear water cutting through mountains at the heart of 2.3-million-acre wilderness named after preservation legend Frank Church. We felt lucky to spot some of the wildlife the area is famous for: mountain goats and otters and bald eagles that soared above us between the pine- and Douglas fir-covered peaks. Early on we also passed a couple of fly fishermen going after rainbow trout in the shallows.

My mind drifted along with our steady flow down the invisible, steep decline of twenty-eight feet per mile, a slope that created the spring and summer fast water and fierce rapids responsible for the river's nickname, The River of No Return; boats could maneuver downstream but not back up. We camped out in tents and spent the next day like the first, letting the ride and sweet-smelling air melt away more of our day-to-day concerns by the mile. At the campsite that night, our guides carefully made a bonfire according to the wilderness rules and my travelers joined me around the fire.

That night, and in many nights to come through decades of women's adventure trips, we shared our personal intentions, beginning the ceremony by passing around a smoking clutch of sage to sweep in front of our bodies as a cleanse and a signal that we were now in a sacred space. I reminded them that everything said in the circle would stay in the circle, so their words were safe. (Stories in this book are shared with their permission.) Holding a stick I had found in the woods earlier that evening, I began by talking about my intention to bring purpose to my own life and bring everyone along for the ride. That was my goal for these trips from the beginning, to engage in a spiritual quest with everyone coming along to reap the benefits of a new adventure on their own spiritual journey.

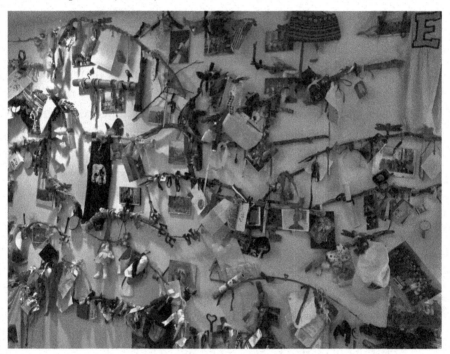

My wall of talking sticks commemorates decades of women's adventure travel. *(Photo: Author's Archive)*

After finishing my little spiel, I passed the stick to the woman on my left who pushed a small, formal-looking piece of paper onto one of the branches. She told us the paper was a leftover

RSVP card from her wedding invitations, now eleven years old. Staring into the fire, she talked about problems she was having in her marriage. *I can't believe I'm saying all this because I haven't told a soul, including my husband, about how scared I am that we're losing what we had.* She cried as she gave us more details about her dwindling relationship and secret fears, and in the end, her desire to work it out. We listened as she poured out her soul. Letting it all out, she told us, helped her see how much she wanted to save her marriage. She felt hopeful about it for the first time. The spark of courage in her voice was palpable—we all felt it.

I sensed that her honesty and willingness to be vulnerable was setting the tone for the evening. The women seemed to relax a bit, stiff shoulders dropping and eyes looking up from the fire to make contact. Our sacred space in the pine-scented air, encircled by ancient trees and the sound of flowing water, felt safer than anything I had known. Maybe the others felt the same.

As I took in the collective sensation that her honesty brought to us, it hit me that this gathering experience accomplished much more than simply daydreaming or journaling about our hopes and dreams could. Sharing our truths—saying them out loud—makes them real. We all have fears, big and small, buried deep or just beneath the surface, but once we express them in the safe space of loving witnesses, they can lose their grip. Our fear of facing facts can turn into a new intention for living. Over the years I gained a deeper understanding of why this ceremony brings a lot of tears: it's liberating to be genuine and to be heard.

The next women to speak in our circle by the Salmon River shared more intentions about their relationships, work, and self-discovery. The peaceful feeling that comes after a good cry had taken hold of the group by the time the stick moved on to the fast-talking New Jersey girl. She stuck a pink grapefruit onto a branch and said, "This has been really deep and everything, but all I want is to lose five pounds before my daughter's wedding." We burst out laughing. Leave it to a gal from Hoboken to provide the comic relief. Some of my travelers feel inclined to dive into the deep end with this ceremony, while others need to keep it simple (not that losing five pounds is easy business). On each trip, no matter where we find ourselves, the circle is ready to hold whatever comes.

On a trip to Mexico several years later, one woman hung a tiny doll's dress on the talking stick and told us her intention was to start a business, a children's clothing store, in her small town in Connecticut. She had thought about it for years but was contending with that all-too-familiar imposter syndrome. A voice in her head kept saying that her lack of training and experience in retail management doomed her to failure. "*You*, a business owner? Right!" the snarky voice insisted. She was convinced that this trip came into her life to shut down that inner critic and help her commit to her dream. Much to her surprise, the simple act of saying this out loud was such a release that she started to cry.

A few months after that trip I ran into one of the women from the Salmon River trip who asked if I had been in touch with so-and-so, the woman who had shared about her marital problems during the ceremony. I hadn't, so she was excited to tell me that she had recently seen her, and she was still married. "She worked it out and she's happy—they're both happy," she said. "Isn't that great?" The woman who wanted to start a business followed through with her intention as well. She's a friend, and I was delighted when she and her business partner invited me to the grand opening of her kids' clothing boutique. As she showed me around the bright little place, she told me that the talking stick ceremony and everything else about those days in the Mexican wilderness empowered her to act. The exhilaration of hiking, bonding with women, and taking advantage of the opportunity to face down her fears stayed with her when she got home, lifting her out of the normal and every day and motivating her to take real steps toward her dream. She said it was all my doing, that I gave her the courage, but I set her straight. I brought her to the canyon, I told her, but the rest was up to her.

Holding the talking stick ceremony on the second night of the Salmon River trip worked so well that I scheduled it in the agenda for night two ever since. By the second evening, we've become acquainted enough to let go of our inhibitions about sharing a personal concern or unearthing a neglected dream. Twenty-four hours of roughing it (in various degrees, depending on the trip) and challenging ourselves on trails or climbs or bikes tends to break down barriers pretty well. On another early trip, for example, two of my travelers bonded the first day over extreme silliness in the small town of Moab after hours of hiking the surreal red rock landscape of Arches National Park. Cheryl Tiegs and my old friend Jodi sauntered into a local cowboy hangout for a lemonade before dinner and, as you can imagine, drew some attention. Everyone recognized Cheryl and assumed, maybe because of her celebrity glow, that Jodi was famous too. She looked a lot like Cheryl Crowe at the time, and as Jodi tells it, the whole place went berserk and people ran up to them with napkins to sign. They both laughed it up as Jodi played along, scrawling a fake Cheryl Crowe autograph while elbowing Cheryl about their secret gag. Later that night, they went to a karaoke bar and the same crowd (Moab's a small town) shouted for Cheryl Crowe—Jodi—to sing. She pretended she had laryngitis and got away with it, and the story of the two superstar Cheryls in Moab lives on in our collective memory.

OFF THE MAIN PATH

Not long after the Moab trip, Jodi joined me on an excursion to Mexico's Copper Canyon, one of the wonders of the world, to scout out as a potential group destination. I needed to check out the little-known hike to the small town of Batopilas near the bottom of a narrow canyon to decide if it was too rugged for the average sneakers wearer. Jodi and I had no idea what we were in for. Thanks to encouragement from Skip McWilliams, an American who had made this corner of North America's largest canyonlands his home for years and who owned a lodge on top and one deep into a canyon in the town of Batopilas, Jodi and I were convinced we could make the grueling trek.

Skip is one of those off-the-beaten track personalities you'd expect to find in a hero's journey-inspired movie script. He'd be the wise man who shows up with his magical gifts to mentor and guide the hero through treacherous terrain and then disappears into the mist. On my many return trips over the years I came to admire Skip's fellowship with the land and its Indigenous Tarahumara owners more and more. He and his Tarahumara outfitting crew were our gatekeepers to the mind-bending, otherworldly scenery of this slice of Copper Canyon, the six-canyon region that dwarfs America's Grand Canyon. If mindfulness is the latest term for the eons-old practice of staying in the moment, Skip is the mindfulness master. Now in his seventies, he recently sent me an email that began, "*These* are the good old days." Exactly. Whether I'm standing on the rim of a gorge in the Sierra Madre's Copper Canyon or stepping into a deli in New York City, every moment is an invitation to experience the wonder of being human. He reminded me, once again, that the miracle of taking a breath, the comfort of peeling apples, and the joy of watching a sleeping child can be peak experiences. For me, honoring every experience with my full attention and no "strings," just simple observing, brings gratitude, which opens the heart. Standing before Copper Canyon's endless landscape of flora, rock, depths, and color instantly ignited a mindful state, good practice for learning to see the glories in the so-called ordinary. To see instead of just look is to behold. Every day in that attitude becomes a good old day.

Jodi and I didn't have any choice but be crystal-clear aware on our scouting trip to the canyons. We arrived at Skip's Sierra Lodge after a long flight to Chihuahua followed by an equally long drive to the lodge a few miles West of Creel, where we entered a phone-, internet-, and electricity-free zone. The log-hewn lodge was lit with kerosene lamps and offered spectacular views that helped shift our mindsets into neutral—ready to move in whatever direction required. The next morning we began the three-day trek down to Batopilas and the river that bears its name, following Skip and our barefoot Tarahumara guides.

They cut the trail with machetes through brush, cactus, scrubby trees, and sprawling agave as we headed along what seemed a meandering course instead of the run-of-the-mill donkey trails Jodi and I had imagined. Maybe this was a shortcut, because I've seen those donkey trails since then—they must have been there all along. Hiking eight hours per day toward a destination we couldn't see until the very end did not feel like a shortcut. But who cares? Copper Canyon brought out the stillness in me in a way yoga or meditation never had. It seemed we were the first humans to step where our feet landed, and maybe we were. This must be how Neil Armstrong felt, I thought as I looked at the loose rock in front of my shoes that no one had laid eyes on before. I got the same feeling when I looked out at the waves of rock and canyons all around us. Before coming here, the Grand Canyon's nineteen hundred square miles seemed gargantuan; now, my mind couldn't begin to process the scope of Copper Canyon's twenty-five thousand square miles. I had to surrender to it along with the sacred impression made by the timeless, uninterrupted patterns of stone and canyons. We could not have rushed if we tried, and not just because of the terrain— the environment held a calm power over us. We just walked and looked and once in a while asked, arms outspread toward the view, "Where are we headed?" Skip would smile and one of the guides would thrust out a finger to point at yet another canyon.

More than once we found ourselves clawing a rock face to make our way along a narrow, nerves-of-steel path with a steep drop-off on one side. "Don't look down," they said. No problem. When the trail got pointy, the Tarahumara guides slipped on sandals made of scraps of tires. They set up camp for us every night and prepared the chickens we helped carry. We city girls named our chickens, of course, and got pretty attached to them. After my first day carrying Shirley by the neck, as instructed, one of the guides made a quick gesture that meant I should twist it. Wasn't going to happen. Skip had to take over, and I didn't get as attached to the anonymous brown hen that had to swing from my grip on day two. That was the day the donkeys sat down.

As Jodi recalled, "They decided, 'That's enough—this is bullshit.' The pack donkeys didn't care what the guide handling them had to say, so all five had to be taken back." That meant half our precious gear had to disappear with them, like makeup and bath salts and a ridiculous number of outfits. We couldn't bear that so we jammed as much as we could into our backpacks, much to our regret at the end of another marathon day on the trail. For Jodi, that was the least inconvenience of the day. Well into the afternoon, she and Rahui, one of the guides she befriended even though he spoke only Tarahumara, were walking ahead of the rest of us when he stopped her and put his finger to his lips—*listen*. All she could hear was the *sssssssss* of copperhead snakes. "There were snakes on both sides," she told me. "Rahui began to walk again, slowly and almost silently. Being barefoot helped, but I had hiking boots on. I don't think I was breathing. All I could do was follow and walk through. You walk through and get on with it."

At the end of the third day we spotted the town of Batopilas that stretches about a mile along the riverbank deep into the canyon. Not long afterward we were checking in at Skip's Riverside Lodge, a restored nineteenth-century merchant's residence built in the heyday of the silver mining era. Sitting in the dining room that evening after a shower and foot soak, I couldn't shake the feeling that no one could ever find me here. I was off-grid, almost off the map, settled on a speck of land at the base of an abyss hidden within the folds of a massive mountain range. To my normal world I was invisible. And to myself I was present for the first time. No connections, no distractions, no expectations. Just one woman and her friend perched on the vibrant, freshwater bottom of the world.

It didn't take long to decide that I would bring small groups to Copper Canyon, but since the hike to the lodge in Batopilas would probably be too challenging for most, I opted to have us driven down and back on the Batopilas Road. We always traveled to Copper Canyon in the fall—summer is way too hot—and loved our first nights on the canyon-rim Sierra Lodge, where our little rooms were heated with wood stoves and fitted with windows that let in the sound of women talking and patting tortillas. Skip and his Tarahumara guides brought us on day hikes through brush that led to rocky outcroppings with vistas of the copper-green canyon moonscape. From time to time we'd glance up at a helicopter belonging to the region's marijuana growers and wonder if we were stepping into dangerous territory, but Skip assured us the "bad guys" would leave us alone, and they always did.

After a few days we made the journey to Batopilas in two bulky Suburbans and road bikes on the roughly paved Batopilas Road. I asked Skip to throw in the bikes to break up the long ride, and he was happy to bring them along. The one hundred-mile, four-hour drive took us up and down canyons along crazy hairpin turns, eventually leaving us six thousand feet lower than where we started up in Creel. We could ride bikes on the easy sections and then pile in the cars when it got too curvy and super steep. Skip strapped a couple of folding chairs to each roof for the brave souls who wanted the best view as the cars crept up and down the mountains. We took turns buckling up for an hour at a time.

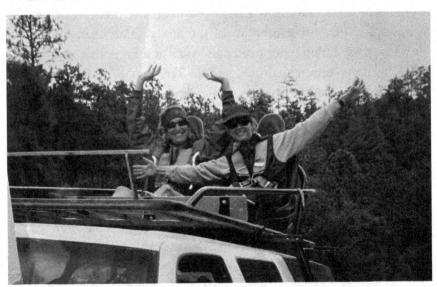

Enjoying the Suburban-rooftop view during a long drive down the Copper Canyon's Batopilas Road. (*Photo: Author's Archive*)

Riding high in the open air I watched the mountain ridges and shadows for pinpoints of white or red that may be the blouse or shirt of a Tarahumara Indian among the cave homes in which a small percentage of families still live (the majority live in small groups of traditional stone or wood houses). The Indigenous people escaped into the canyons when the Spanish colonizers came into the area in the sixteenth century. The bits of Tarahumara history I learned from Skip on my first visit inspired me to learn more, and I passed along recommended reading to the women who signed on for my trips to make their experiences richer. The world marvels at the Tarahumara for their resiliency as a people and their phenomenal skill in endurance running, which they developed as persistence hunters who could outrun their prey. In the past few decades, anthropologists have learned more about the social and spiritual interconnections in long-distance running, persistence hunting, and ritual dancing (a feat of constant, quick footwork lasting at least twelve hours) in Tarahumara culture. The extreme conditions of the Sierra Tarahumara mountains make Tarahumara running stand out among that of other Indigenous running cultures, and for Tarahumara men, women, and children, running is about much more than sports, hunting, or staying fit:

[Tarahumara] running is spiritually meaningful, a form of prayer, a symbol of the journey of life. It is impossible to measure the extent to which these attitudes and beliefs help motivate runners to dig deep and find the strength to keep going for long distances that many people from other cultures find impossible to imagine.[1]

---

1   Daniel E. Lieberman et al., "Running in Tarahumara (Rarámuri) Culture, *Current Anthropology,* Vol. 61/3, June 2020, https://www.journals.uchicago.edu/doi/10.1086/708810

Being in the Sierra Tarahumara's Copper Canyon in the flesh, as your body registers the steep inclines and ascents of the rough terrain, makes it truly impossible to imagine running in this landscape for hours on end in bare feet or minimal sandals. My mind spins with questions when I'm there: What would it feel like to achieve a runner's high on a steep, rocky, uncut path? To dance nonstop for twelve hours? What would my body be capable of today if I had been taught to connect with the Earth through distance running and dancing from childhood? These thoughts, which stay with me long after I return home, are one more gift of the Sierra Tarahumara.

On each trip our small groups have met several families, including those belonging to our guides, who lived in small villages near our hiking paths. I brought them gifts each time— clothes, coloring books, toys—and loved watching the children grow one year at a time. Some of us wanted to take the Batopilas Road down to the village on the river every time, and the ride back up was always as white-knuckle as the trip down. On one trip, Jeri from Florida begged us to let her sit on the roof chair the entire way back. Entranced by the scenery and focused on the hairpin turns, we forgot all about her. Three hours into the journey it dawned on me and I blurted out, "Oh shit, Jeri's still up there!" The driver stopped and we rushed out to take a look. She was perfectly fine, grinning from ear to ear as she gave us two thumbs up.

Copper Canyon is more on the adventurer's radar today than it was in the 1990s when Jodi and I first explored it. It's still a primitive destination, which is what attracted me in the first place. I was looking for hard-to-get-to, non-flashy places off the beaten path. You never know where a half-page article in a beaten-up hiking guide is going to take you...in this case, it dared me to take a step off the main path, as Chippewa poet Margaret Noodin puts it.

GETTING THE VIBE RIGHT

Our early adventures introduced us to ethereal worlds like Copper Canyon and unexplored spaces within ourselves that seemed eager to find a voice in our circle around the campfire. There were less subtle lessons too, like the night we had an unexpected shock in Santa Fe, New Mexico. My intuition kicked in big time during that trip, telling me something was off. I couldn't figure it out right away, but the evidence kept growing. Eventually I realized the mix of personalities didn't quite fit—the temperaments of a few were too unsettling to make the group coalesce. I went with the flow anyway, trusting that things would work out as needed in the bigger picture. What worked out was bad...and I blamed the chemistry.

After spending a couple days camping near Bandolier National Park, we checked in to our lovely hotel outside Santa Fe and went into town for dinner. When we returned to our rooms, they'd all been ransacked. The doors were hatcheted to pieces and everyone had been robbed. Several women had their cameras, film, jewelry, and money stolen, and some took it better than others. I was just grateful no one got hurt. As Marjorie and I held hands in my room, staring at my ripped up bed and empty wardrobe, we shook our heads and managed to feel grateful that it wasn't worse. "It's just stuff," I said, and she agreed.

A few others in the group weren't as philosophical. Some showed their true colors, which clashed with the ideal I had managed to create with previous groups. I wasn't looking for angels, just people who were open minded and at ease enough to get along with anyone. I failed with my selection for that trip, and we all paid the price. This trip, the only one so far in which something went wrong, was my big learning experience. Getting robbed anywhere is such a violation, but this offered a chance for me to take stock of how differently people handle it. I thought a lot about what I could have done differently to avoid what happened. Maybe I should have thought long and hard about any potential personality tweaks that would create a less-than-easy-going vibe at times. The robbery may have been an extension of that disharmony—I was responsible for not having the chemistry right, and something had to give. Or maybe I didn't leave a big enough tip when the staff took our luggage, so they weren't mindful about our rooms while we were gone. Both reasons seemed plausible, and I blamed myself for each of them. I'm still in touch with a lot of people from that Santa Fe trip and we sometimes talk about how tough it was to settle in to a vibe that just didn't sync.

The silver lining—there's always a silver lining—was my renewed respect for my intuition. That night I made a pact with myself to listen to my intuition when arranging trips to ensure I would get the chemistry right, and in the process I've been able to rely on it in every aspect of my life. The silent nudges I easily dismissed in the past I now consider potent, indisputable guidance designed to steer me in the direction that will create the best outcome for all concerned. The more you act upon that guidance, the less hazy it feels the next time it appears in the back of your mind or the middle of your gut. It becomes normal, habitual, and extremely helpful. When I talk about this with women on our travels, I find that most of us share a strong reliance with our intuition in this, the over-fifty stage in our lives. I see it as another gift that comes with maturing into our fullest selves. That's why I include listening to your intuition in my list of principles to live by, culled from my experiences as a woman, daughter, sister, wife, mother, and adventurer of the world and the soul.

Seven Principles for Trekking Life with Grace

1. **Nix the Competition.** It doesn't matter if you're out front, in the middle, or at the back of the trail, because the journey is about how alive and grateful you are in every step.

   My friend Marjorie recalled the moment during one trip in which she chose to abandon her competitive edge for her own good:

   > One of the most physically challenging trips was in the Canadian Rockies, where we were in our crampons and all roped in, climbing very high. I was scared. I was in the second group, and at one point a girl in the first group slid down a bit. Erin looked back at me and tears were coming to my eyes. I thought, I'm not doing this. I stayed behind, looking out at the tree line, basically contemplating my navel while the girls went ahead. For me that was the right move at the right time. All the things we learned on the climbs became a metaphor for life: when you're on a ridge, you look out, not down. In life, you look forward.

2. **Walk with Integrity.** As the saying goes, "Integrity is doing the right thing, even when no one is watching." To have integrity is to walk life with honesty, sincerity,

truthfulness, humility, and a sense of responsibility—not just toward others, but also toward yourself.

We all live through adverse times and traumas, and how we navigate through those daggers defines our integrity. Our responses guide our evolution as either authentic, compassionate people or those who keep trying to swim upstream. My fellow traveler Judy described how getting out of her comfort zone helped her develop an inner core of personal integrity:

> In Cambodia, we had guides with machetes cutting through the jungle wearing flip flops and smoking cigarettes. I looked down and saw blood on my socks because I'd been bitten by leeches. Just part of the experience. These trips push me out of my shell a little bit. We're a team, and that's part of the beauty of it. There's no whining allowed; you just go with it. It is what it is, and you make the best of it and go forward. That's such a good life lesson. When you come home and you have issues, you think back about how you climbed that craggy rock and know you can do this other thing, you can figure it out.

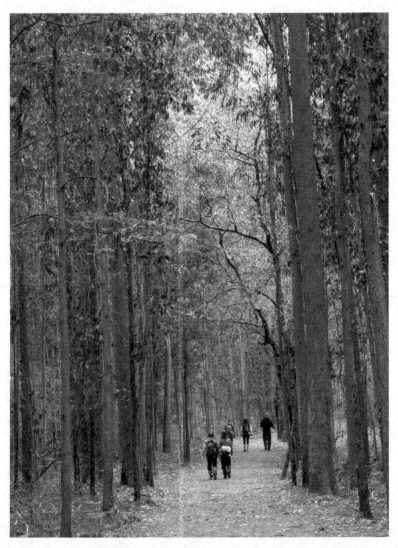

Walking with humility beneath a towering canopy on Spain's
Camino de Santiago. *(Photo: Judy B. Nussenblatt)*

3. **No Judgement.** Judging another doesn't define them, but you. You can never walk someone else's path, so drop your assumptions, avoid gossip, and meet others with an open heart.

Travel adventurer Ruah experienced a transformation when she let go of her knee-jerk first reactions about a fellow traveler:

> I was having such a negative emotional reaction to this one woman, and later, on another trip, I learned that she had a past that hadn't always been pleasant, like many of us. In reality she is an amazing, lovely, caring person who I came to respect and admire. I learned that when you delve deep, listen, and open up you become nonjudgmental, which creates a bigger community for you filled with very interesting people. I am now able to listen openly and judge less quickly.

4. **Start with Effort, Finish by Grace.** Once you've prepared all you can for something, relax and leave the rest to the universe. Grace is the ultimate "doing" that takes no action on our part—it just comes. When we get out of the way and invite grace, things fall into place and amazing connections and "coincidences" appear.

My email to my Sports Travel Adventure Therapy clients on March 19, 2020, described how my decision to not schedule any trips for 2020 "coincidentally" turned out to be the perfect plan, since (as we would all learn early in the year) the coronavirus pandemic would prevent travel: *Six months ago, I decided to take 2020 as a sabbatical "clarity year" off from travel. Little did I know, the world would join me. Last year at this time (March 2019), I was putting the final touches on the two extraordinary trips we experienced together in 2019—one to Italy and the other to Japan. I'm so grateful we were able to experience these journeys together before world-wide travel came to a standstill, but I'm also feeling sadness for our wonderful Italian guides and inspiring Japanese pilgrims on the sacred trails of the Kumano, and how they are surviving the crisis and what's next for them. Like we've reminded each other at countless STAT ceremonies, though we have tough times, they always are the times that teach us how to connect with deeper meaning and purpose in our own lives. We learn. We grow. We heal. And eventually, we thrive. This too will pass. Be patient. Let's manifest our intentions together to heal the world.*

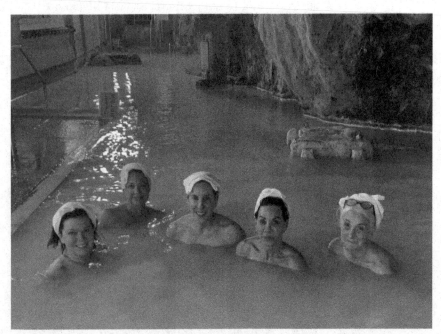

Cleansing our souls in an onsen, the Japanese ritual hot springs bath. *(Photo: Author's Archive)*

5. **Mark Your Words.** Begin each day breathing in your power words, pulling them up through the center of your body until the last one hovers above your head. My words are *clarity, consciousness, equilibrium, effort, grace, intention, integrity, love.* The last word rains down to embrace me in a gentle calm. Sitting before my altar that holds a statue of Ganesha, the remover of obstacles, I meditate on these words as they rise through my body and then feel strong and grounded the rest of the day. When you set positive intentions for yourself with a ritual practice such as this and with consciously intending your highest good, you're ready for anything.

Shannon's first opportunity to join an adventure trip came during one of the most challenging moments in her life, and her brave decision led to a powerful experience in letting go:

> One of my friends got me invited on the trip to Tasmania, but a few months later I was diagnosed with breast cancer. Deciding whether to back out or not was a challenging decision, but I wasn't stage four or anything. I was just wrapping my head around the cancer word. My doctor said, 'Go. I can't see you for a month anyway, so calm down and have a good time.' It was the best decision ever. I definitely was not the healthiest person on the trip because I'd also had a knee replacement the previous year. And at home, raising my family, I was always the planner, always in charge, so letting somebody else plan this trip, feed me and shelter me, was an interesting experience in letting go of

control and of needing to lead and be first. I decided to follow way behind and soak up the nature. I knew I was not in control of the trip and not in control of this stupid cancer. I let things go and got calm about it. I think that new calm was big. It helped me heal when I went through chemo. Lying on the couch, I let it go.

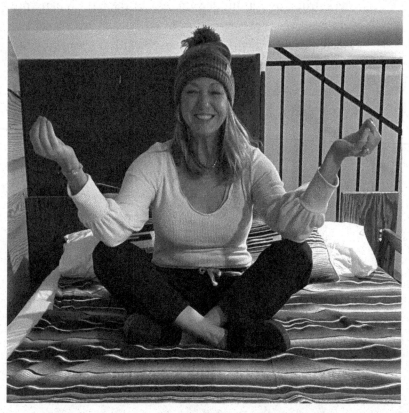

Beaming, cancer-free Shannon on a later trip to Ojai, California. *(Photo: Author's Archive)*

6. Love, Honor, and Obey Your Intuition. I believe that nature never wastes a thing, so the automatic guidance system we call intuition must have evolved for a reason. Intuition is our sixth sense, the natural "knowing" that goes beyond the other five. Why ignore such a gift?

Steve Jobs believed in having "the courage to follow your heart and intuition,"[2] Einstein said "intuition, not intellect, is the open 'sesame' of yourself,"[3] and poet and novelist Robert Graves called intuition the "supra-logic" that allows us to "leap straight from the problem to the answer."[4] Psychologist Carl Jung went all out with his definition: "What some people call instinct or intuition is nothing other than God. God is that voice inside us which tells us what to do and what not to do. In other words, our conscience."[5]

I learned to value my intuition the hard way after a disastrous trip to Santa Fe confirmed my sense that the chemistry of my group was all wrong. I have trusted my intuition much more seriously ever since and acted upon its wisdom. Give your inner voice a chance next time it whispers to you. If you do, you will develop a finer ear for its nudges, hunches, and gentle prodding—all designed for your highest good.

---

2   Cal Newport, "What Steve Jobs Meant When He Said 'Follow Your Heart,'" April 5, 2015, https://calnewport.com/what-steve-jobs-meant-when-he-said-follow-your-heart/

3   William Hermanns, *Einstein and the Poet: In Search of the Cosmic Man*, Branden Books, 2011.

4   H.A. Dorfman, *Coaching the Mental Game*, Lyons Press, 2017.

5   Carl Jung Depth Psychology, May 7, 2020, https://carljungdepthpsychologysite.blog/2020/05/07/carl-jung-on-intuition-and-intuitives-anthology/#.YLmtFC1h0iM

7. **Embrace Community.** Our hardwiring for loving relationships and social bonds shows up in how these experiences affect our physical, emotional, and mental health. COVID-19 taught us many things, including how tough it is to be isolated from our friends and loved ones. Many of us became sick at heart as well as sick with the virus. As we celebrate our ability to gather together again, I am reminded that loving connections start with our ability to be vulnerable and face ourselves and others with authenticity. At the heart level, self-discovery changes everything, as my friend and former neighbor Susan M. discovered during an earlier time of crisis in our country:

> When 9/11 hit, it woke me up in a way I had never thought about. I was going through life before 9/11 kind of blindly thinking I'd do in my life "just what you do." I thought, I'm going to be married, have my three kids, a white picket fence, and this is going to be my life. Then 9/11 happened and something shifted in me. I saw the world fall apart before my very eyes and decided I didn't want to die without knowing what love is. My life could end in two seconds, and I realized I hadn't discovered love yet. That was the main thing I worked on in all of Erin's trips. It was almost like the four characters in the *Wizard of Oz*, each searching for something that, in the end, they saw was in them all along. I went on the *Wizard of Oz* adventure through Erin's trips to discover what was inside me the entire time. The love.

☙

FOR REFLECTION

1. How does the closeness you feel with one person—your partner or best friend—compare to the connection you feel when you're with a group of friends? Are there topics or experiences you share with your partner and not in a close group, or vice versa?

2. What is the most challenging physical experience you've had (a sport, on vacation, moving, etc.)?

3. Which of the Seven Principles of Trekking Life with Grace do you feel you already incorporate most fully in your life? Which do you think need more attention?

4. Write up a personal example of how you have experienced/expressed each principle.

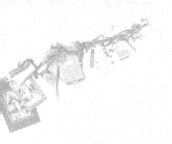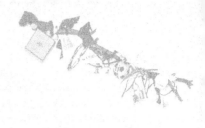

PART II

TREKKING LIFE WITH GRACE

As we grow old, the beauty steals inward.

—Ralph Waldo Emerson[1]

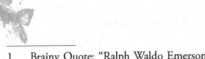

---

1   Brainy Quote: "Ralph Waldo Emerson," https://www.brainyquote.com/quotes/ralph_waldo_emerson_104255

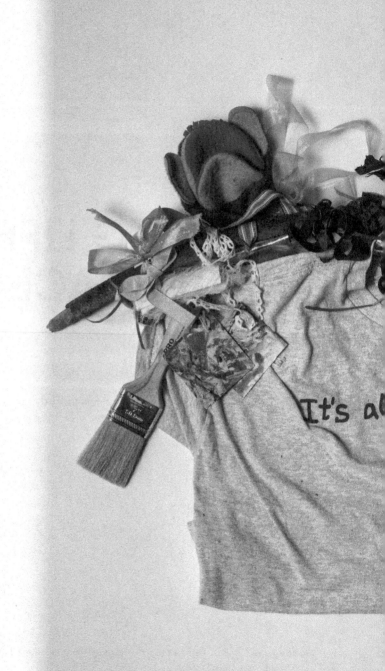

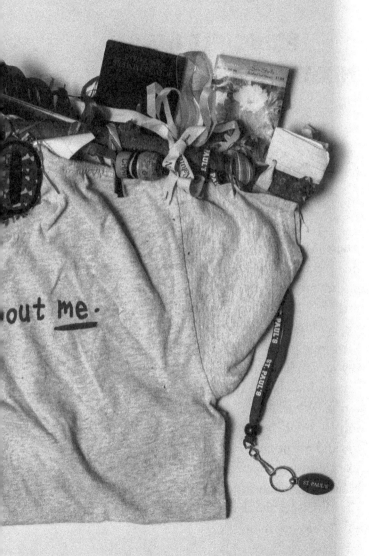

CHAPTER 4

PRINCIPLE I:
NIX THE COMPETITION

Comparing yourself to others is an act of violence
against your authentic self.

—Iyanla Vanzant[2]

I LOVE MY FRIEND MARJORIE's view of competition. On our trips, she gets better and better at mountain biking, and her pride in that accomplishment is not about passing up her fellow travelers (which she may or may not do) on a twenty-five-mile ride, but about pushing her limits and showing herself that she's capable of more than she thought she was. She says it's all about the mindset: "You tell yourself, 'I can do this; I can certainly try. I may be in the back of the line, but that's fine. People are stronger than I am—that's fine. What matters is that I'm here. I'm doing it.'" Marjorie's only sense of competition is with herself as she faces down her fears and old notions of herself. In the process, she feels her insignificance in the scheme of things as she rides across an astoundingly beautiful plain in front of a mountain range. The setting is a gift of perspective that hones life down to its essence; we are part of all this, not masters of it.

---

2   Iyanla Vanzant, Twitter, September 3, 2012, @Iyanlavanzant.

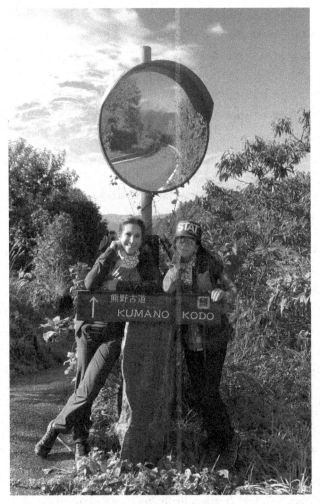

Marjorie and I on the Kumano Kodo, Japan's ancient
pilgrimage trail. *(Photo: Judy B. Nussenblatt)*

The competitive drive to outdo others fades away in moments
like those. Most of us were probably brought up to believe that
success, and the happiness that is supposed to come with it, only
arrives for those with a competitive edge. Americans, especially,

seem conditioned to believe that life is about the survival of the fittest—if I push harder than others, I'll move up a spot and someone else will move down—it's a zero sum game of winners and losers. My generation was taught that this is how evolution works in the natural world. But it's not true. In recent years the real story of species survival has come to light and blasted through the myth about competition as the end-all to success and survival. Competition has played some part in our survival as a species, but it's not the whole story. Humans have survived and thrived because of our knack for cooperation. As Douglas Rushkoff, author of *Team Human* explains:

> Individuals and species flourish by evolving ways of supporting mutual survival…. Survival of the fittest is a convenient way to justify the cutthroat ethos of a competitive marketplace, political landscape, and culture. But this perspective misconstrues the theories of Darwin as well as his successors. By viewing evolution through a strictly competitive lens, we miss the bigger story of our own social development and have trouble understanding humanity as one big, interconnected team…. Evolution may have less to do with rising above one's peers than learning to get along with more of them.[3]

My wake-up call on Kilimanjaro, when I accepted the fact that I couldn't finish the climb and felt okay about it, was a turning point in helping me develop an even healthier competitive nature. Growing up as a cheerleader and sports lover, I felt more competitive with myself than with others. Sure, I wanted to be one of the winners who made the squad, but most of my competitiveness was aimed at challenging myself to be the best

---

3   Douglas Rushkoff, *Team Human*, Norton, 2019, p. 11, 13.

I could be. I've since learned that this approach to competition has a name, *constructive competition*, which sees competing as a fun approach to self-development rather than a nail-biting way to perform better than others. People who hold a constructive, positive attitude toward competition are all about improving themselves, and competition becomes a way to measure how far they've come. *Destructive competition*, on the other hand, is driven by a need to be dominant. This negative aspect of competition shows up in people who need to overcome rivals in order to feel good about themselves.

We've all got our own style, and that includes what kind of motivation feeds our competitive outlook. Positive competition comes from *internal motivation*, the desire to do something for the pleasure and adventure of it. Call it getting out there and walking, writing, doing your job, learning, or playing an instrument for the sheer satisfaction of doing it and getting better at it. As a teenager I felt internally motivated to master the gymnastic moves of cheerleading and later on to excel as an aerobics teacher and outdoor adventurer. That's different from competition driven by *external motivation*, which wants to engage in something not for its own sake, but just as a means to an end. It's a craving to win instead of an itch to play.

At the extreme end, when a competitive spirit becomes hypercompetitive, a person needs to compete and win at any cost because their sense of self-worth depends on it, and things can get aggressive. The opposite of that attitude was all over the news in the summer of 2021 when Naomi Osaka, the number-two-ranked tennis player in the world, showed us what positive competition looked like. The twenty-three-year-old tennis star chose to skip the French Open to take care of herself, sending shockwaves through the sports world. What kind of superstar walks away from one of the most prestigious meets in the game?

One who plays to master the game for herself, according to an Instagram post she addressed to a fan: "You're on your own path and don't look at what other people are doing for comparison. Your only competition is yourself. You're the only person living your life and walking your path so treasure that."

Naomi Osaka's humble attitude and kindness in taking the time to comfort a stranger reminded me of the anti-competitive message taught by Phakchok Rinpoche, a Tibetan Buddhist teacher from Nepal. He teaches a simple method of turning away from our competitive nature that starts with setting aside five or ten minutes to sit and

> feel fortunate, feel meritorious, feel very thankful or very content with what you have. And after that, you can rejoice with what other people do, what other people enjoy, when they have success, and when they have a good time. Simply rejoice and feel content, no further than that. This will bring some happiness that you won't get from spending 8 hours being competitive. Just 5 minutes of feeling fortunate and rejoicing in other people's actions brings happiness.[4]

This brief meditation sounds simple, but gratitude is a powerful emotion. Rinpoche's advice to start with gratitude and then feel joy for someone's good fortune can shift your foundations. Focusing on another person's accomplishment instead of letting your mind race with comparisons, frustration, or envy is a practice in mindfulness. Buddhist teacher Jack Kornfield's Eastern perspective describes mindfulness as a "loving awareness" in which simply being here and now evokes a quality of resting in

---

4   Phakchok Rinpoche, "Dealing with Your Jealous and Competitive Mind," *Tricycle*, August 17, 2016, https://tricycle.org/article/dealing-with-your-jealous-and-competitive-mind/

love so that "love and awareness are actually the same." Eckhart Tolle, with his books *The Power of Now: A Guide to Spiritual Enlightenment* (1997) and *A New Earth: Awakening to Your Life's Purpose* (2005), also introduced this idea as an alternative to our competitive approach and worldview. Tolle doesn't use the word "mindfulness," however, because he does not want to emphasize "mind." Like Kornfield, his message is about moving beyond "thinking" to enter a peaceful state that is only aware of the present moment. He calls this "being in the Now," letting go of the mind's chatter, obsession with the past, and judgements (about oneself and others) and instead being fully aware of what *is*, right now:

> The only place where you can experience the flow of life is the Now, so to surrender is to accept the present moment unconditionally and without reservation. It is to relinquish inner resistance to what *is*.... Acceptance of what *is* immediately frees you from mind identification and thus reconnects you with Being.[5]

Tolle captures the sense of being "beyond mind" that I and many of my fellow travelers have experienced in nature. We find ourselves lost in the breathtaking view, scents, hawk cries and birdsong, wind in our faces, and awareness of our tensing muscles, and there is no room for thoughts. Tolle says that being out in nature can indeed make us "naturally free of the stream of thinking, and those are the most worthwhile moments in your life." When we're walking through a forest, hiking, or climbing a mountain, he says, we are completely present "and suddenly you feel so peaceful." Why? Because "in that moment you are conscious and consciously perceiving, but not thinking."

---

5   Eckhart Tolle, *The Power of Now: A Guide to Spiritual Enlightenment*, Namaste Publishing, 2004, p. 206.

Like all wisdom teachers, Tolle and Kornfield want us to consider that peacefulness can be our new normal. Habits like negative competitiveness can fall away when we take time to stop and simply witness what's in front of us. I've done this on the golf course, watching a friend's swing as she follows through with a beautiful combination of strength and fluidity. In that moment my mind is far away, leaving me free of envy or any restless comparing of scores. The game is much more fun that way.

Artists too can trade in their competitiveness for a state of peaceful mindfulness, even in situations that normally ignite high anxiety. Concert pianist Josh Wright, for example, who has won top prizes in several competitions, is a longtime fan of Eckhart Tolle. He had just read *The Power of Now* for the second time when he competed in the 2013 Heida Hermanns International Piano Competition, and he started the day by listening to a couple of his favorite chapters of the audiobook. He showed up to the event, he said, "in a mental state of utter calmness," feeling not only peaceful, but more alive than any time he could remember. Backstage, immediately before his entrance, he listened to a meditation from the book that simply said, "I believe, I trust, I let go." As he wrote in his blog:

> As I walked onto the stage, it felt as though I was more aware of my breathing, sitting down on the bench, the scent of the piano (Steinways have a very specific scent...), lifting my hands to the keyboard, and then just letting go.... It was as if there was a wall between my thinking and my playing... I was enjoying myself, but it wasn't because I was performing. It was because I had total acceptance of what was happening. It didn't matter any longer how I played, but rather that I was sharing what I loved with the audience, and more importantly,

enjoying what I loved doing. I finished playing, and it suddenly dawned on me how well I had performed.[6]

Josh won first prize that day and credits his experience of "unconditional self-acceptance" as one of the most important lessons of his life. For him, performing is no longer about competition or analyzing every move he makes. "Whenever I approach the stage now," he wrote, "it is with love towards myself and the audience, rather than criticism of myself and hope that the audience will like what I do."[7]

I've seen a similar letting go of self-criticism—and the deep change it brings—on some of my trips when a traveler pushes herself a bit too far. One year, my friend Donna had a tough time at the beginning of our hike on a section of Spain's Camino de Santiago. She had put inserts into her hiking boots without taking out the original ones, which messed up her balance and left her with such an aching back she could barely walk. I told her she was welcome to ride in the van, our backup vehicle for situations like this, but she refused. She didn't want to give up. By dinner time she was in excruciating pain, and two women in the group, Nevine and Abbie, both yoga instructors, offered to help. This time she let go of her pride and said yes.

"They used every piece of furniture as a prop," she recalled, "and twisted me in positions I didn't even know my body could do." The next morning she felt better and was ready to get back on the trail, but with a different intention. Instead of trying to keep up, she stayed in the back with Judy, who always walked behind everyone else to take photos. At that slower, uncompetitive pace,

---

6   Josh Wright, "Letting Go." February 12, 2014, https://www.joshwrightpiano. com/blog/letting-go

7   Josh Wright, "Letting Go." February 12, 2014, https://www.joshwrightpiano. com/blog/letting-go

Donna got the message she felt she was meant to learn: "Slow down and take it all in. It's the journey, not the destination. It took my body breaking down to let me see that you don't have to be out in front." In that new state of mind, Donna's second-day hike was filled with mindful moments of watching sheep graze and cats peek out from charming doorways. Thanks to the yoga experts' generous help, she told me, her heart was filled with gratitude, which gave the trip a spiritual dimension for her.

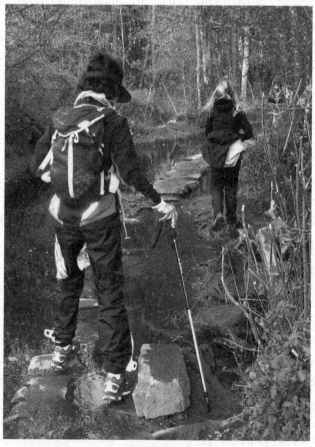

Donna (foreground) taking it slow but happy on the Camino de Santiago. *(Photo: Judy B. Nussenblatt)*

Those yoga instructors, Nevine Michaan and Abbie Galvin, are my longtime friends and very well known throughout the global yoga community. Nevine, with whom I have studied for more than twenty years, created Katonah Yoga, a technique that embraces the all-is-one wisdom of Taoism as well as concepts from sacred geometry, mythology, and other esoteric fields. Nevine is more than my teacher; her outlook and brilliant way of making yoga—and life—mystical and practical at the same time have had a deep influence on my own worldview and the way I carry myself.

Katonah Yoga is based around three principles, starting with the concept of threeness, or the trinity, as the mediating/harmony-making factor in everything. In the mystical sense, one plus one doesn't equal two, but three, because something new, a miraculous third thing, is born from an interaction. That third thing could be a baby born of a man and woman or a new idea that springs from and builds upon previous ideas. The second principle says that the universe has pattern, and patterns reveal a foundational intelligence behind everything. The third principle observes that repetition holds the potential for insight. Repeating yoga poses, a meditation technique, or scales on the piano leads to development and learning that result in new insights.

Nevine believes that being mystical, or looking into the deeper meaning of things, makes good sense for anyone who wants to enjoy life: "It's very practical to be mystical," she said, "because the world is very big, and it's much more fun if you have a big mind for it."[8]

Nevine's philosophy, like herself, is non-competitive. She believes that yoga is not about performance, but about informance. We explore our bodies inside and out to understand

---

8   Centre Yoga, "Nina Reis," https://www.jpcentreyoga.com/nina-reis

ourselves, where we fit, where we feel best, where we are most alive. All the yoga poses are meant to fit; it's not to be forced. Yoga practice is about the ebb and flow. No one's body is created equally, so certain poses hurt people. A pose should not hurt. There's no such thing as no pain, no gain. That's a fallacy. If a pose hurts, it's informing you that your body doesn't want to go here, not today. Maybe you'll feel better with it and be more flexible tomorrow. It's an internal game, a spiritual practice. It's not a sport. Power yoga? There's no such thing—that defeats the whole purpose. Yoga poses are supposed to inform your body what the infinite possibilities are, both physically and mentally. Yoga is not a sport, it's a practice.

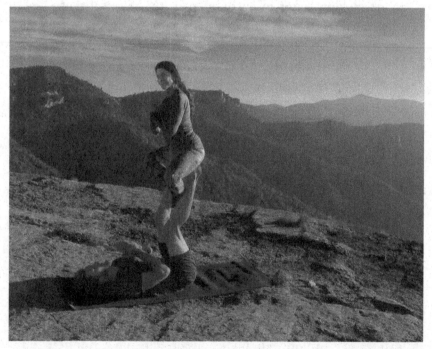

Getting acrobatic with morning yoga on a mountaintop in Spain. *(Photo: Judy B. Nussenblatt)*

Abbie expanded yoga lovers' access to Katonah Yoga by opening her own yoga venue, "The Studio," in New York City. She infuses her yoga practice, teaching methods, and lifestyle with her mentor Nevine's philosophy, carrying out her personal life mission to help others "live a richer, more informed, satisfying life."[9] In her home practice book for Katonah Yoga students, Abbie reminds us that shifting the mind inward into the body's intelligence through yoga brings more physiological wellbeing that in turn impacts our psychology. "When we consciously and consistently turn our attention to an interior enterprise," she writes, "we can better process our thoughts, feelings, impressions and debris from our daily lives." This makes a daily yoga practice "a technique for self-revelation, self-discovery and self-awareness."[10]

Because it's a practice, like life is a practice, yoga has taught me a lot about competition. We're all practicing; nothing is perfect. My competitive edge has softened into a more interior intention to be the best person I can be at any given moment, in any situation. I want everyone to win and to succeed. If they succeed, that doesn't mean I can't.

Another STAT traveler, Julie, experienced a deeply personal kind of success during our second trip along the ancient Camino trail. In 2016, eight of us hiked the Portuguese Camino, where we joined walkers, bikers, and even horseback riders heading north along the Atlantic Coast just like Queen Isabel did in the 1300s. This walk through terraced fields, lush forests, plenty of vineyards, and peaceful villages represented everything STAT is about…a sacred bonding journey. Walking nearly fourteen miles together all day every day was the ultimate bonding experience. We shared our stories while still taking time alone to reflect on

---

9   Abbie Galvin, "The Studio," http://www.thestudio.yoga/abbie-galvin

10   Abbie Galvin, *Katonah Yoga Home Practice,* The Studio, 2018, pp. 3–4.

ourselves. Julie came with a heart full of hope for her son who would soon be released from prison. If all went well, she and her husband would have their beautiful son back, clean and sober.

Her son had suffered from addiction since his teen years when he was prescribed painkillers after having his wisdom teeth removed. Percocet led to OxyContin and then heroin, and Julie and her family watched him diminish from a handsome, robust, six-foot-tall young man to an ashen, one-hundred-twenty-five-pound addict living on the street. More than once he had over-dosed and was brought back to life by emergency teams armed with naloxone, and he continuously stole from his family to feed his habit. The worst point in Julie's life was when she and her husband had their son arrested for stealing and had to testify against him in court. He was sentenced to three-and-a-half years in prison, where he began to heal.

A month before he was to be released, Julie went on the Portuguese Camino trip. Her mother had recently died, so she brought her ashes along to scatter along the sacred ancient trail. She also brought a photograph of her son and photos given to her by people who asked her to pray for them or their children as she walked the hike. Two pictures were of children suffering from addiction and one was of a friend in her early forties diagnosed with stage four cancer. "Her outlook was grim at the time," Julie said. "I tied photographs on the talking stick when we began our journey, and at every church we visited along the route I prayed for them and sprinkled a few of my mother's ashes. I don't believe in coincidences, so I know my mother was with us because every time I spread her ashes, no matter what time of day, the church bells rang."

Julie went on the trip to gather her strength and become grounded with women she hoped would be along a spiritual path.

"Holding up those photos of those beautiful people struggling in their lives and being around all these women just felt right and whole," she said. When the group reached the end of their journey at Finisterre, "the end of the world," a rocky point jutting into the ocean on the Spanish coast, Julie sprinkled the last bit of her mother's ashes and said, "Mom, you made it to the end of the Earth." But that wasn't the end of her story. "When my son was released, he was a new man," she said, "and he has stayed sober and been rebuilding his life since then." Over time, the other two addicts also got clean, and her girlfriend's cancer went into remission and she has been completely healthy for the last year and a half. "All four were my own little miracle," Julie said.

I love reading about miracle and success stories. There is room in the world for all the winners. Who among your friends is winning on their spiritual path, in their family life, their work? Just look around; there are so many winners. Everybody just wants to find joy. My trips with women teach us to be trusting— we're all human and everybody's going through the same thing. Being together for a few days or a couple of weeks breaks down barriers. A lot of stuff comes up when you're hiking or biking and giving it your all, even your need to compete. And that can change everything.

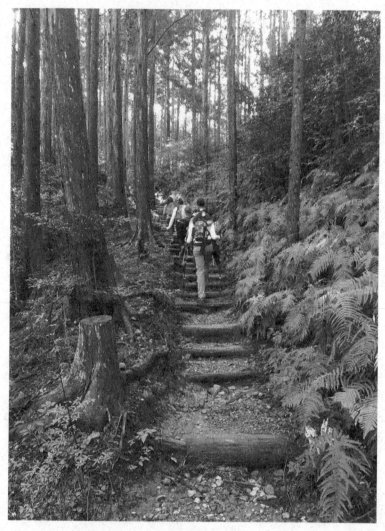

Japan's wondrous Kumano Kodo Pilgrimage Trail. (*Photo: Judy B. Nussenblatt*)

ↂ

FOR REFLECTION

1. Do you consider yourself a Type "A," competitive person or more laid back? How do you think your close friends and family would describe you?

2. What activities in your life spring from your internal motivation to bring yourself pleasure, fun, and satisfaction?

3. Who is the most competitive person you know? Without judging, does their competitiveness seem to have a more positive or negative impact on their life?

4. Recall a time when you felt you were immersed in the calm, deeply focused "flow" of an activity, when your actions felt effortless, and time seemed to stop.

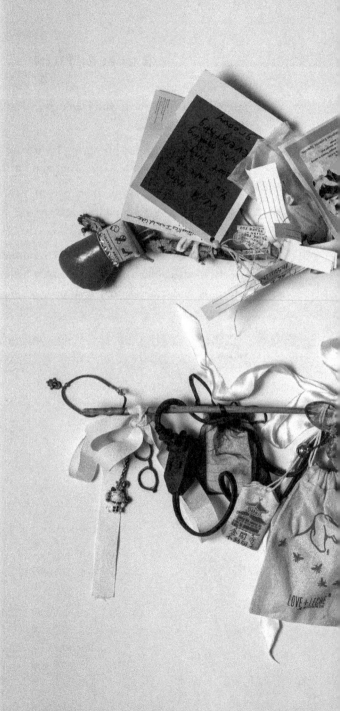

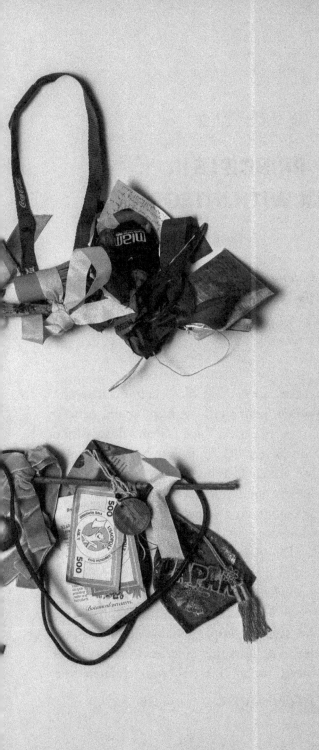

CHAPTER 5

PRINCIPLE II:
WALK WITH INTEGRITY

Three things cannot be long hidden:
the sun, the moon, and the truth.

—GAUTAMA BUDDHA[1]

ABOUT THIRTY-SIX YEARS AGO, I was in a euphoric state after having my first baby. On phone calls with my mom, between my details of our son's every perfect fingernail and flossy wisp of hair, she told me Dad was very sick. In fact, unbeknownst to me and maybe her, he was gravely ill as his cancer had spread. Mom probably thought she was doing the best thing by shielding me from what was going on at such a vulnerable and precious time with my new baby, but the fallout of her lack of transparency haunts me to this day. Dad passed away before I had time to say goodbye, and I had no real closure with him. Mom could have let me be the judge of whether or not I should rush to Miami to be at his side. Instead, I missed out on what could have been a milestone in my life, saying a proper goodbye and being present at my father's death. At least this experience came with an important lesson—never try to "protect" your children from

---

1   N.K. Sondhi, *Small Things Matter Most*. General Press, 2019, p. X.

life's painful truths. Not telling the truth will most likely cause more suffering. I believe it's best to respect people's right to know and to deal with life's tragedies in their own way. As Thomas Jefferson's adage goes, "Truth will do well enough if left to shift for herself."[2] When we allow truth to run its course through us, we become more human and more whole.

My women's travel adventure journey has always been founded on helping women become the best version of themselves, because when we are the most whole, we have the most to give. The small but epic moments of awe and transformation that come with exploring nature and coming out of our routines change us. I'm not changing the world—I don't have a cure for cancer—but I believe I touch women's lives for the better. Part of this involves offering them ways to give back and connect with the places we visit.

A few years into my women's travels I was fortunate to meet a woman who helped me add this philanthropic element to our trips. For the past dozen years, thanks to the truly inspiring change-maker Lydia Dean, co-creator of the GoPhilanthropic Foundation, STAT has given back to each community we visit and at every opportunity provides funding for various critical needs around the world. Lydia's foundation empowers small grassroots organizations—from a child rescue group in Nepal to an early education organization in Guatemala, for example—to stand on their own by supporting their work with small to midsize grants.

My travel company recently supported one of Lydia's partner organizations in India devoted to protecting women and children's rights. Lydia told me about a request from the organization's founder, Anuradha Bhosale, who fights tirelessly against

---

2   Thomas Jefferson, *Notes on Religion* (1776), published in *The Writings of Thomas Jefferson: 1816–1826* (1899), edited by Paul Leicester Ford, v. 2, p. 102.

injustices to women. Anuradha had humbly told Lydia that her night shelter was in critical need of their very own transport, a *tuk-tuk* (auto-rickshaw), so they could not only react immediately to women in need of protective services but also collect anything they need on a weekly basis. STAT provided the funds for the vehicle and I was moved to see Lydia's photo of them giving it a traditional puja blessing before it hit the road.

Anuradha and her team, devoted to women in crisis, strengthen my commitment to give women opportunities to bond and challenge themselves beyond their comfort zones to become their best selves. Giving back in a meaningful way has made each STAT trip even more fulfilling and meaningful for me and all my fellow travelers. Like me, many of them had not considered looking into how to support specific needs of a community until later in life. I didn't grow up in a philanthropic family, so my giving back developed out of my own searching and purpose. After STAT was running full gear, I felt a sense of responsibility to support the remarkable people we met who gave so much to us. With that intention in mind, lo and behold, I crossed paths with Lydia. Years later, my women travelers' philanthropic activities continue to connect us deeper to the land we meander and celebrate so actively. Giving back, like exercise, generates a strong sense of purpose and we experience more gratitude, love, hope, and community.

Lydia's path from being an American expat wife and mother raising her family in Europe to launching a foundation gave her a solid, feet-on-the-ground understanding about the art of giving. She learned from experience that the most well-intentioned Westerners need to find their own integrity and authenticity before they can genuinely help anyone else around the world.

NO MORE ASSUMPTIONS

Following an inner call while raising her two young children, Lydia signed up to spend two weeks teaching English at an orphanage in the Chennai district along the Bay of Bengal in eastern India. She felt ready to do her part in a corner of the world with many needs, but after a day or two of working with fellow volunteers and the bright, eager children, she wondered how much two weeks offering English could really accomplish. Those like her who wanted to spend time doing good somewhere had wonderful intentions, but as Lydia continued travelling she realized that the key to making a real impact was not to rush in with preconceived ideas about how to fix things, but instead to support what people were already doing to improve their lives and communities. She eventually teamed up with two kindred spirits to cofound GoPhilanthropic and partner with local organizations, raising money and people-power to support their homegrown projects like installing wells, building school computer labs, contributing basic resources to orphanages, and getting mobile libraries on the road.

Lydia told me that she developed this support-the-grass-roots perspective of philanthropy the hard way. "Wanting to make a difference under the assumption that we actually have answers for people from the other side of the world who have walked a very different life is very presumptive," she said. She recognized that the typical Westerner's approach was top heavy with a sense of superiority. When Americans and others come in with their power and privilege, thinking they know what is best for the community, they start off on the wrong foot, and as a result, not a lot will change. Lydia and her cofounders turned that around by creating a dignified way to help people who have found solutions for their issues but need tools and funding to develop and grow.

Their ethical approach didn't happen overnight. "I fumbled my way through building something that was better," Lydia said. "I made a lot of mistakes. But when you surround yourself with people who know better than you, you have an open space where you're learning from others how to create something good." In her experience, this kind of work begins with examining oneself.

"When we peel away all the layers of ego that normally drive us and function from the source we all share, we do not see people as poor or underprivileged," she said. "We see ourselves in them. That was a real turning point for me. Seeing these magnificent changemakers, very rich in courage—there was no room for pity there." Working from that open, selfless space, she said, allowed a sense of authentic justice and harmony to automatically emerge. "That natural harmony happens organically," she said. In her memoir, *Jumping the Picket Fence*, Lydia describes the point of her philanthropic work and its ultimate reward:

> We continue to offer journeys where people can sit face to face with the true changemakers of the world. I have come to appreciate what happens in these moments as nothing short of sacred. Travel has represented the magic road to my own personal connection and understanding of humanity—facilitating this for others, and seeing the resulting beauty unfold, is a true joy.[3]

I admire Lydia for her willingness to follow her intuitive sense that volunteering to teach English to impoverished orphans isn't enough, and maybe not on track at all. The people in that district knew what and how to teach those children, and they just needed more resources to do it. Lydia looked further and learned

---

3   Lydia Dean, *Jumping the Picket Fence: A Woman's Search for Meaning*. Lydia Dean, 2015.

she had to find her own core so she could work from there, and in that process of challenging her assumptions and conditioning she uncovered her authentic self. She is a wise woman with remarkable integrity.

While Lydia's foundation supports people doing the good work they know their communities need, I use travel to help women uncover their strengths and sense of connection with their bodies, nature, the land, and other people. I am always amazed to see the effect of these experiences on women as they become more whole versions of themselves and take all that creative energy and compassion out into the world. My friend Susan Barron, an artist whom I've known since college and our semester together in London (and who took the talking stick photographs shown throughout this book and on the cover), changed the direction of her life after our trip to Cambodia in 2009. Lydia arranged for us to visit a school, and the day we arrived changed everything for Susan.

BACKPACKS AND PTSD

Riding in a van with our guide on the edge of Phnom Penh one morning, a dark hill in the distance caught our attention. Getting closer, it turned out to be a mountainous garbage dump crawling with trucks…and children. Our guide explained that the dump hired kids to search for recyclables, a dangerous business in such a filthy and unstable setting where they ran the risk of slipping beneath the rubbish or getting run over by a truck. According to our guide, some of the poorest children in the city took the job to scratch together money to help their families who lived on the sidewalks or outside the city. Collecting bits of plastic and metal didn't earn them much, and the last thing they could afford was school supplies.

Those kids who felt they could spare the time attended a nearby school launched by a local woman, Phymean Noun, who grew up in the killing fields during the Khmer Rouge genocide and managed to get an education and graduate from high school. Lydia arranged for us to meet Phymean, who by that time had become an internationally known hero for her work as a teacher and provider for these children through her foundation, the People Improvement Organization. We didn't know a lot more about her at that time except that her high school diploma had earned her a job in the United Nations office in Phnom Penh, and after building a secure life with money in the bank, she walked away from it all to help the poorest children in the city. Education had taken her out of poverty and opened many doors, and she was committed to giving these children the same chance.

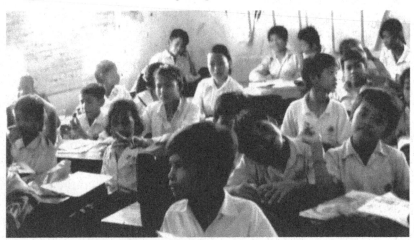

Boys and girls in one of Phymean Noun's classrooms in Phnom Penh.

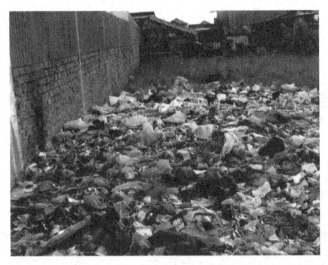

A nearby garbage dump where children searched for recyclables. *(Photos: Judy B. Nussenblatt)*

After ten minutes of watching the kids pluck glass and other trash, we asked our guide to turn around and take us shopping for school supplies to bring to Phymean during our visit. When we returned an hour later, our hearts were bursting as we met Phymean and about fifty of her students and handed out backpacks stuffed with notebooks, pencils, paper, rulers, and crayons. The children handled these items like priceless jewels. Our donations made a difference, but Susan could not let go of the fact that we were one small group doing one seemingly small thing. As she tells it, that day at the dump triggered an idea that changed the course of her life:

> For the rest of the trip I kept feeling that this was such an unsustainable business model. When is the next group of crazy American women going to stop and buy school supplies, when a continuous group of kids will be at the garbage dump every day? They had no clothes, maybe

an old tattered t-shirt, that's it. The only way out was an education. And this couldn't be the only place this was happening. I thought of the one-for-one concept of Toms Shoes, where for every pair purchased the company donates a pair to a child in a low-income country. I drew up a business model on the plane on the way home for a business that would do the same with backpacks filled with school supplies.

Susan launched the Pencil Promise that same year and made backpack deliveries to children in Cambodia, Laos, India, Cuba, Indigenous tribes in Kenya, and elsewhere. She patterned the deliveries after our women's adventure trips, bringing groups of women and/or families to hand deliver the backpacks to the children and walk them into their schools. They would then explore the area, such as having meals with families and, in Kenya, taking a safari in one of the national wildlife parks. "I took my boys when they were done with school and we went as a family," she told me, "and we will always cherish those experiences. The travels were incredibly meaningful to me and my family and were a direct result of that one STAT trip to Cambodia. I really feel we made the world a better place, a little bit at a time."

A few years later Susan started to focus her attention on people in need in the United States, particularly military families, after learning about their financial struggles. "I was introduced to some women who lived on an Army base near me and they said they had no money for school supplies and barely enough for food," she told me. "Their husbands were on multiple deployments and they couldn't live on what they made, especially in the New York metro area. One woman had five kids and only the oldest got a backpack—the others got a pencil in a plastic bag." Susan reacted to this situation by setting up barbecues and other events for families, where she and her team would deliver backpacks. She made the events even more special by rounding up local sports celebrities to come along and sign notebooks for the kids.

At one of these events, the military wives told her that their husbands had come back from multiple deployments, having survived combat in both Afghanistan and Iraq, and killed themselves on the streets of their hometown. Susan dug into the shocking facts about post-traumatic stress disorder (PTSD) and military suicides, which were occurring twenty-four times a day across the country (a number that persists in 2023). She delved into the issue with her camera, traveling from state to state to photograph veterans and learn their stories about the invisible scars of war.

To raise awareness about the PTSC epidemic, Susan created mixed media portraits to illustrate the veterans' experiences in their own words and collected them into an exhibit entitled "Depicting the Invisible." The exhibit continued to tour the country in 2022, and film director Robert Rizzo produced a documentary short[4] about Susan's project that has won multiple awards.

Meeting the children in Phnom Penh sparked a creative fire in Susan that sent her on a new path as an artist and humanitarian. She has used her abundant gifts to help make school a reality for children and to create art that makes the invisible wounds of war visible to all of us.

---

4   Susan J. Barron, "Depicting the Invisible," Susanjbarron.com, 2021, https://
     www.susanjbarron.com/documentary.html

ERIN LEIDER-PARISER

ANOTHER GOOD SIDE OF GIVING

Blending a charitable piece into my trips takes the experience to a new level and often inspires women to do philanthropy on their own. Gina Berlin, for one, began including giving-back elements in her personal travels after participating in our group trip to Cambodia in 2009. When her son was old enough to appreciate a long trip, she took him and her nephew on a five-week hiking and biking trip to Asia, complete with scheduled giving trips to local organizations. In Tokyo, for example, they donated to and spent a half day visiting Kidsdoor, an organization that helps lower-income families get a high-standard education. During their jaunt to Bali, they did the same with the Sea Turtle Society—supporting and learning about the importance and relevance of the group's work to Indonesia's ecology (who knew there's a dark trade in sea turtles?). Gina put these and other excursions into their trip to broaden the boys' understanding of their own situation and country as well. "I always say to Jake, when you get up in the morning, the first thing you should do is kiss the ground you walk on, be grateful for all the many opportunities you have, and do not take the U.S. for granted because a lot of countries, as he sees and hears when he travels, can only dream of the life that we have in the U.S."

Lydia's initial guidance for the Cambodia trip gave me the tools I needed to seek out fitting ways to give in the places we later traveled. While planning a trip to Croatia, for example, I learned that a village school on the island of Korčula needed computers, so I arranged for the group to purchase laptops we could personally deliver to the children. The kids were so excited to see us and had prepared a song; we could tell they had worked so hard and were proud to show what they could do. Afterward they took us to a small restaurant where women had spent more than a day preparing a feast of local dishes. The image of the children's joyful faces never faded as the twelve of us sat at one table, enjoying seafood dishes like black risotto with squid and garlic. Being able to come together later and share our asanas after experiencing a beautiful connection with the children and women at the restaurant only enhanced our gratitude for our own blessings in life.

For a trip to Myanmar, I collaborated with a travel agency to host a traditional Buddhist ceremony—let's call it a Buddhist b'nai mitzvah—for seven boys and three girls. Entering the monkhood is a rite of passage, and they study and prepare for this day as my boys did for their bar mitzvahs. Invitations were sent out to the entire village, and all of us dressed in traditional Burmese garb to be part of the procession carrying silver bowls with flowers and the novices' new robes. Talk about the rewards of connecting; we felt honored to be part of such a profound occasion. Providing the funds to make the event happen for the entire village, as it ideally should, made us bond with the people and the place in a way we never imagined and have never forgotten.

The good feeling of giving, doing the right thing, treating people with dignity and respect—living with integrity—seems to have a biological purpose. Our body chemistry rewards us when we serve each other, so nature sees a value in it. Scientists have found that giving of ourselves, such as donating to charities, releases pleasure-producing endorphins in the brain and gives us what they've dubbed a "helper's high." Giving also decreases stress, which has a positive impact on health and longevity. We also benefit from stronger social ties when we give and are given back in return. This back-and-forth experience expands our feelings of trust, which in turn increases our bonds with others and improves our health. Being generous makes us feel closer to people; the act of giving makes us perceive others in a more positive light.[5] I see the "warm glow" of giving on my trips as my fellow travelers connect to the people we meet and to each other. Generosity on any scale, from offering a kind word to cashing in your savings to build a school next to a garbage dump, heals the world.

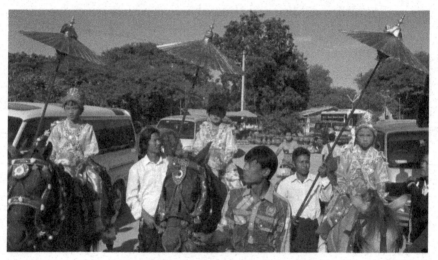

Children parading in their ceremonial costumes during the ceremony we hosted in Myanmar. *(Photo: Author's Archive)*

HONESTY

While honesty is the best policy, at times it may be uncomfortable to tell the honest truth when someone could feel slighted or offended by it. In my business, however, a lack of honesty could do real harm. After the Santa Fe fiasco early in my travel adven-

---

5   Jill Suttie and Jason Marsh, "5 Ways Giving Is Good for You," *Greater Good: Berkeley,* December 13, 2010, https://greatergood.berkeley.edu/article/item/5_ways_giving_is_good_for_you

ture days, I was more serious about getting the group vibe right. From the start, I also carefully measured up the physical demands of each trip and did not allow women who weren't up to those challenges to attend. I'm honest about telling women that a trip isn't for them if I know it's too rigorous or just not a good fit— my honesty is based on caring for their welfare.

Some of my fellow travelers have shared how these adventures have brought up issues about their honesty with themselves. Cheryl Tiegs told me about one trip in which she completely made up her little speech during the talking stick ceremony. The incident baffled her so much that she recalled her discomfort around it years later. "I don't know why I did this," she said, "but one time they went around the circle and came to me, and I said, 'You know, my life is so happy. I have nothing to complain about or even talk about.'" Meanwhile, she said, her life was a mess:

Why would I do that? I kept looking around at all these girls and thought, why am I lying to these lovely ladies who could help me? I always wonder why I did that, because they were just there to help, to love. I've pondered that a lot because my life was probably at one of the lowest points. On every other trip I was quite honest in the stick ceremony. But everything going on at that time must have been too overwhelming to talk about.

Being honest in the ceremony is critical, because first of all, whatever the problem, you realize you're not alone. You're not the only one; you're not the first one. Generally people have had experiences very much like yours so they can talk to you about how they felt. It's such a good way to get through something, such good therapy, because you walk in for breakfast the next day and someone will tap you on the shoulder and say, 'I went through that and this is how I felt.' It helps enormously. Why I didn't do that when I needed to most, I don't know. There was no judgment from anybody. All other times, the ceremony was an amazing way of opening your heart and having others listen who might help, or might not, who knows. It's a way of healing.

Cheryl wasn't honest with the group on that trip, at least during the talking stick ceremony, but her instinct to be truthful with me about that moment, knowing I would write about it, shows that her sincerity and humility are intact. These virtues, closely connected to honesty, show up as measures of our integrity.

Life coach and sociologist Martha Beck has an interesting definition of personal integrity as the state of being whole and undivided, like we were when we were born. As we conform to society to be well-behaved and make rational choices, our wholeness is split up and we become a divided self. A young man, for example, who wants to major in literature in college may be stymied by his parents who convince him to get a business degree as the route to a more "secure" career. Later, he's never truly happy in his work. When we bury our sense of purpose, Martha says, it is still there, "like a flower trying to grow through toxic sludge."[6] We can make our way back by realigning with our truth.

Fellow STAT traveler Sonia Gliatta grew closer to her truth after a transformative experience during her first STAT trip. As she integrated her new awareness into her work, she felt a deeper satisfaction with life.

---

6   Martha Beck, *The Way of Integrity: Finding the Path to Your True Self,* Penguin, 2021, Ch. 1.

TRUTHFULNESS, SINCERITY, AND HUMILITY

Sonia's first trip with us, a voyage to the jungles of Brazil in 2008, put her more in touch with her spirituality and how to bring it into her life through compassion and service. We began that adventure by hiking six to eight hours for two days to reach our main camp, where we met up with two grandmother shamans who had been preparing a space for us to perform cleansing rituals with water. "There was something about these two women on that mountain," Sonia recalled. "They made it possible for you to let go and trust whatever prayer they're saying or ritual they're conducting—you just accept it and embrace it." She said that the spirituality of those events went beyond her experiences with religion. "At the time I considered myself very Catholic, but this had nothing to do with being Catholic, Jewish, or whatever else."

The shamans gave each of us handmade satchels filled with little crystals, jade, agates, and other stones. For the first cleansing ceremony, they led us deeper into the jungle to an area with waterfalls cascading over large boulders. The grandmothers took off their clothes and went into the water, and we did the same. For Sonia, the ritual opened up something inside that filled her with joy. After one of the prayers, I was standing next to her on a rock where a small waterfall rained down on us and she felt an extreme release. "I could only laugh, cry, and smile," she said—"it was incredible. Something spiritual happened to me at that moment. I felt totally changed." After coming home to New York City from the trip, she got more serious about her yoga and meditation. She had viewed yoga as a good stretching exercise, nothing more, but now looked deeper into the spiritual aspect of the practice.

Sonia soon felt drawn to volunteer at a hospital in the Bronx, working with women cancer patients on simple yoga poses they could do without getting on the floor. "We did chair yoga and breathing practices," she said. "Everyone was so grateful for the time you took to sit with them. Some were not familiar with yoga and started out with a little stretching exercise. Then they started figuring out it was about a little more than that, and that it helped them, so they stuck with it. It was very gratifying to see them transform through some of these classes."

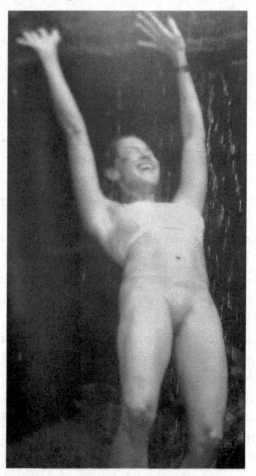

Sonia's transcendent waterfall moment in Brazil. (*Photo: Judy B. Nussenblatt*)

Sonia's spiritual awakening, fed by grandmother shamans and a mysterious waterfall, inspires me in its humility and sincerity. When she tells her story, I see her life like a movie that gradually blooms from black-and-white to technicolor. Her experience in walking with integrity is a gift for her, her family, her patients, fellow travelers, and all of us.

CR

FOR REFLECTION

1. Whom in your circle of friends, family, or work do you especially admire for their integrity? On the other hand, has anyone in your circle done something that shows a lack of integrity?

2. If you are a parent, which children's movies do you appreciate for their characters that express honesty, compassion, and generosity?

3. Have you ever been dishonest with yourself? Why?

4. Make a list of ways—other than a financial donation—you could offer assistance/be of service to a person or organization in your community. Have you done any of these actions? If not, circle the one you would like to do first.

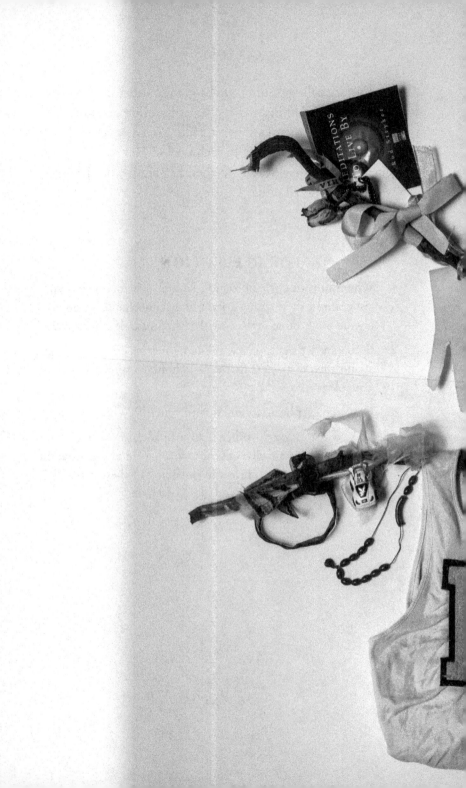

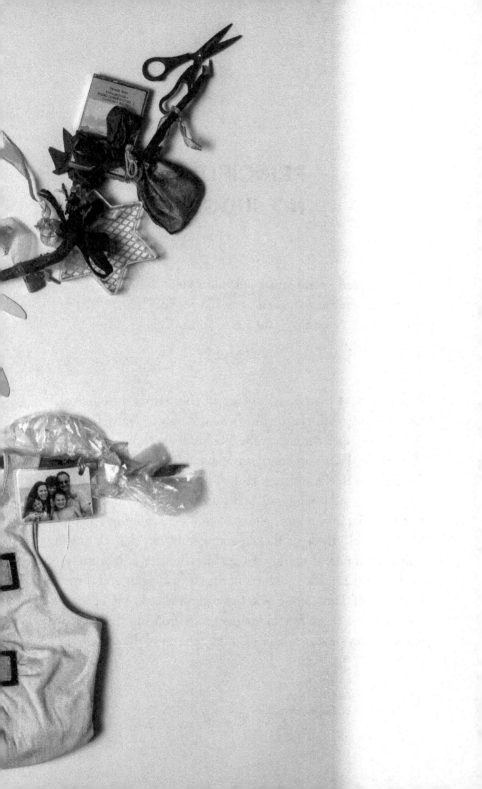

CHAPTER 6

PRINCIPLE III: NO JUDGING

Kindness toward others and radical kindness to ourselves
buy us a shot at a warm and generous heart,
which is the greatest prize of all.

—ANNE LAMOTT[1]

RIDING A BIKE IN THE dark blasts all your senses into high alert and fills you with the thrill of the unknown. We were gliding through another tunnel on the Via Verde de la Sierra, or Green Way, in Andalusia in southern Spain. Mile after mile of abandoned train tracks and tunnels had been transformed into a scenic walking and biking trail, and some tunnels were long enough to require lamps on our helmets. Soon after entering one pitch-black tunnel, my light flickered and went out. I kept moving, following the faint red circle of a bicyclist ahead. My attention fixated on the sudden coolness of the air rushing by and the mineral scent of damp stone. After two good whacks my light came back on, but those few moments of confronting the unknown without slowing down kept me high the rest of the day.

1   Anne Lamott, *Hallelujah Anyway*, Riverhead, 2017, p. 12.

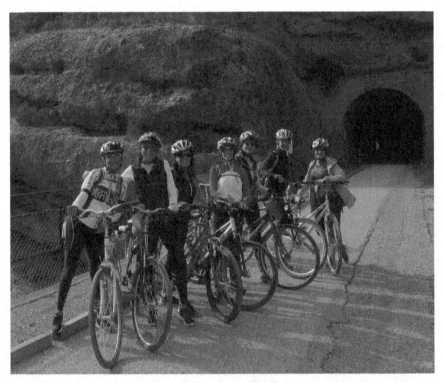

Biking through pitch-dark tunnels in southern Spain with lamps
fixed to our helmets. *(Photo: Judy B. Nussenblatt)*

That incident reminds me of the feeling I usually have when
meeting someone for the first time. Curiosity comes first, with
no assumptions or judgements. I say I "usually" come to encounters in this way, but no one's perfect. At least I've approached new
people from this perspective for as long as I can remember and it
has become part of my nature. I bring it to my adventure travel
groups, not to intentionally model it, but to be as authentic as I
can be, never letting a "leadership" role veer me from my center.
As I mentioned earlier, I've learned that being judgmental doesn't
say anything about the person you target, but says a lot about
you. This is a lesson we learn along the way.

In the Jewish religion, gossiping—a way to spread judgmental talk—is a serious no-no. Slandering or speaking badly of someone is a sin called *lashon hara*, "the evil tongue." I was brought up with the saying that gossip kills three people: the one who speaks it, the one who listens, and the one who's the subject of it. If someone around me starts in on a piece of gossip, I don't engage. At times a woman traveler may point out, say, that it was rude for a woman in our group to only eat a salad and handful of nuts when our guides or hosts spent hours preparing a meal for us. I let that go—both the complaint and the salad-eating behavior. No one knows the whole story behind such actions, and the point of our group travels is to be open and learn from nature and each other. I remind myself before every trip that the journey is the destination, and our travels are an opportunity to bond with people, to open their hearts, to laugh out loud and cry together, to be a shoulder, an ear, and just there for one another without judgement. Women blossom in these moments. They tell me they open up more in a circle of fellow travelers huddled under the stars in a strange land than they do with their own spouses because they know they won't be judged or challenged, simply heard.

Opportunities to put our judgmental inclinations aside are everywhere. Screenwriters and other storytellers are genius at tapping into our instinct to judge and then forcing us to step back. I think of how disgusted I was by Tony Soprano's violence and lack of empathy in scene after scene in "The Sopranos" until a flashback would show his narcissistic dad doing something just as bad. Those moments showed me that Tony's biggest role model didn't give him much to work with. That didn't make me forgive Tony for his actions, but it did make me more empathetic toward him as an emotionally damaged person. Good stories are based on complex characters like Tony who remind us that there's always more going on below the surface.

I love a story that messes with my knee-jerk reactions by thrusting me into a new impression of a character. It's a reminder that life is not black and white and our autopilot tendency to judge is just a remnant of our wiring for survival. Part of becoming a mature person means being less reactionary, and I have an opportunity to do this whenever something unexpected pops up during an adventure trip, such as the power outage that hit us one evening in Hvar. After an afternoon romping around the lovely vineyards, lavender fields, and beaches of this idyllic island off the coast of Croatia, we were getting cleaned up to go to the hotel restaurant for dinner—and the lights went out. Standing in my room in my bathrobe, I wondered how we'd get a meal or do anything the rest of the night, since the juice for running the faucets, stoves, and everything else that makes a restaurant or business run had gone kaput.

Then I just went with it.

I remembered that our guides knew the island like the back of their hands and would always have a plan B. Sure enough, they soon arrived with salad and pizzas from the only restaurant set up to bake without electricity and we dined in the stunning hotel lobby by candlelight. The bar was open, the mood was high, and we danced on the table with our Croatian scarves flying. It turned out to be the best night of the whole trip.

No one in our group blamed the Croatian authorities for not getting power back all night or the hotel manager for not having a butane stove on hand, although we heard some grumbling from other guests. I felt a little bad for those guests because their choice to blame and criticize rather than accept "what is" prevented them from enjoying a night like ours. As ecologist Sven Erik Jørgensen wrote, "Having the courage to move beyond 'fight or flight' reactions to other people, we can shift toward a predominance of relations more aligned with 'tend or befriend.'"[2] In other words, the mature way is to follow the Golden Rule and not mistreat or judge others, just as we don't want to be mistreated or judged.

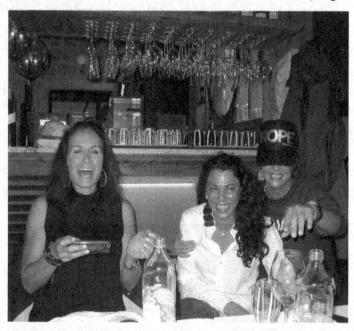

Belly laughs in the Croatia hotel bar as Beth (left) reads her latest story inspired by the day's events and our swarthy yoga instructor. *(Photo: Judy B. Nussenblatt)*

Yoga is part of my maturing, helping me live in the moment with no expectations or judgments. I have a good idea what to expect from my body before I start my morning asanas, but if a joint is not as supple as the day before, I don't force it or blame myself for whatever may have tightened me up. In a class or group, yoga is never about judging others' poses or strength. If you find yourself in a yoga class that isn't calm, unrushed, or

---

2   Sven Erik Jørgensen et al., *Flourishing Within Limits to Growth: Following Nature's Way.* Taylor & Francis, 2015, p. x.

compassionate, fold up your mat and walk away. Yoga is about cultivating inner stillness, and a judgmental attitude toward yourself or anyone else in the room has no place in it.

Rigid approaches are also out of sync with the spirit of yoga, as I learned thirty years ago when I studied Jivamukti yoga, the most popular form of the practice in New York City at the time. The sessions were stringent and hard line; if you didn't measure up to their exacting standard of each pose, watch out. New students or those who weren't flexible enough to fully stretch, for whatever reason, would hear about it. If you needed to bend your knees a little while doing the downward dog, the teacher would stride over and say, "Straighten your knees!" The vibe was tense as teachers demanded we do the archetypal poses and do them "right." Who needs that?

When I started to study with Nevine, she said, "If you can't straighten your knees, bend your knees." Her approach ran opposite to Jivamukti, instilling in us that yoga isn't rigid. It's about listening to your body. Once I started with Nevine and Abbie, my yoga practice went to the next level and I learned that no body is built the same. My experience with meditation went through a similar route of starting out with a more fixed approach than I use today.

I began daily meditation about ten years ago by taking a course in Transcendental Meditation (TM®), in which I received the mantra that would be the basis of my practice. Everyone who learns TM gets a mantra they keep entirely secret—no one knows my mantra except me and the teacher who gave it to me. The TM method, brought to the U.S. by Maharishi Mahesh Yogi (famously known as the Beatles' guru), is straightforward, calling for two twenty-minute sessions of sitting meditation each day. I was taught to repeat my mantra in my mind and let my thoughts flow in and out without lingering on them. The key is to always go back to the mantra, gently, no pushing, and not get frustrated when thoughts keep wanting to take center stage, as they always do. I respected this ancient form of meditation and soon experienced its promised benefits of feeling more energized and refreshed after each session, but I couldn't always do two sessions per day. There is no slacking on this part of the method—TM is a two-sessions-a-day deal. I found this too rigid. Consistently doing the morning session was easy because I could shape my schedule around it, but once I started my day my time often got away from me. I found myself not being able to fit in those twenty minutes or forgetting about it completely, and if I tried to do a session after dinner, I often fell asleep. On days I skipped the second session, I felt guilty and judged myself as an undisciplined slouch.

After a few years of being hard on myself, I learned that periods of meditation have a cumulative effect. You get the same benefit from doing a few minutes in the morning and whatever you can fit in later in the day because the practice works on you over time. I didn't have to be so rigid in order to feel like I was actually "a meditator." A handful of teachers I found through books and online talks and podcasts changed my thinking, letting me know a less structured way was okay and no one was judging me. I could be gentle with myself and make my practice truly my own. Since then I sometimes meditate with my mantra and other times follow guided meditations by teachers I have come to love. Some mornings I sit in my room in front of my Ganesha (remover of obstacles), outside on my terrace facing the mountains, or on the living room floor with my pup sound asleep in my lap. I've relinquished the idea that there is only one way—life shifts, things change, and you embrace it and move on.

Mindfulness and meditation are always opening doors in my everyday life, making it possible, for instance, to come across the work of a teacher just when I'm ready for their particular message. Three living teachers who have been especially influential to me are Tara Brach, Sam Harris, and Joe Dispenza. Each of them point us to the natural capacities we have to live in the way we are destined to live, with a core of inner peace that brings insights, compassion, and happiness. For psychotherapist and Insight Meditation teacher Tara Brach, mindfulness is directly related to a nonjudgmental mindset that she calls *radical acceptance*. She explains that the two aspects of genuinely accepting ourselves and whatever is happening in the moment are "seeing clearly and holding our experience with compassion."[3] When we see ourselves, imperfections and all, with clarity, and then make choices from a compassionate heart rather than self-judgment, we feel free and become open to new options waiting to "open before us."[4] Remembering Brach's acronym RAIN helps me quickly move into a mindful state if I feel tempted to judge myself or someone/something else:

> **R**ecognize what is happening;
> **A**llow the experience to be there, just as it is;
> **I**nvestigate with interest and care;
> **N**urture with self-compassion.[5]

Neuroscientist and teacher Sam Harris writes that "the traditional goal of meditation is to arrive at a state of wellbeing that is imperturbable—or if perturbed, easily regained."[6] This is an ideal way to live, but there's more. Harris explains that the deeper meaning of meditation has to do with embracing the understanding that all is one. Even our sense of a personal "I"

---

3   Tara Brach, *Radical Acceptance: Embracing Your Life With the Heart of a Buddha*, Random House, 2004, p. 27.

4   Ibid., p. 29.

5   Tara Brach, "Resources—RAIN," https://www.tarabrach.com/rain/

6   Sam Harris, *Waking Up: A Guide to Spirituality Without Religion*, Simon & Schuster, 2014, p 44.

can fade away in meditation, leaving us perceiving "the totality of experience." Harris writes that because this perception is "inherent to the nature of our minds," it is a natural state, part of being human.[7]

Another of my favorites, researcher and teacher Joe Dispenza, has explored the harmony, or coherence, that appears in the brain when we meditate. Like any inward contemplative practice, meditation brings body and mind to the present where they aren't bogged down by stressful thoughts or feelings about the past or future. In a meditative state, he says, we are capable of doing extraordinary things like rapid healing. Instead of being in fight-or-flight survival mode, we channel all that energy into creating new brain pathways that put the body's natural abilities into hyperdrive. Like Brach, Harris, and other science-minded spiritual teachers, Dispenza not only describes what our lives can be like, but how meditation and mindfulness practices get us there. When we meditate, for example:

> More individual [brain] circuits start communicating in an orderly fashion and process a more coherent mind. Your awareness shifts from narrow-minded, overfocused, obsessive, compartmentalized, survival thinking to thoughts that are more open, relaxed, holistic, present, orderly, creative, and simple. This is the natural state of being we are supposed to live by.[8]

Quiet, undistracted listening to talks, podcasts, and books by these and other teachers as part of my spiritual practice nourishes my heart and soul. They are gifted with teaching what seems to be mindfulness on steroids, taking us as deep as we can go at any moment.

---

7   Ibid., p. 124.
8   Joe Dispenza, *Breaking the Habit of Being Yourself*, Hay House, 2012, p. 209.

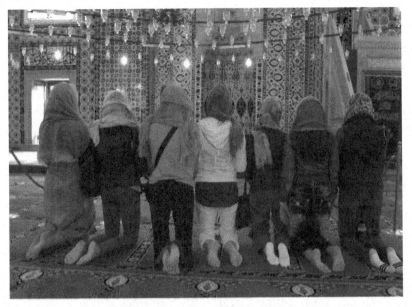

When in Turkey... Praying in one of Istanbul's three
thousand mosques. *(Photo: Judy B. Nussenblatt)*

INDIGENOUS WISDOM

I am writing this at a time when the country is painfully divided.
Lines have been drawn that are affecting people's lives far beyond
the discomfort of disagreeing (even silently) with someone's poli-
tics. As this rift grows, I try to prioritize what connects us, which
is always more profound than what divides. Other cultures,
much older than our European-settled U.S., put connectedness
first, from a spirit of cooperation to a fundamental belief that
their lives are bound in a natural harmony with nature. A message published by group of Indigenous leaders in 2020 describes
this lived philosophy:

> Indigenous cultures often share the view that there is no
> good, bad, or ideal—it is not our role to judge. Our role

is to tend, care, and weave to maintain relationships of balance. We give ourselves to the land: Our breath and hands uplift her gardens, binding our life force together. No one is tainted by our touch, and we have the ability to heal as much as any other lifeform.[9]

This notion of balance and connection extends to the Native American cultures' understanding that what goes on inside us is reflected in how we act. Something out of whack in our mindset, such as self-judging, leads to acting that way toward others, and the hurt goes on. Larry Merculieff, an Aleut born on St. Paul Island in Alaska, explains the layers of this understanding and how it is lived in his culture:

According to many elders, relationship is what life is all about. With a proper relationship to oneself it is easier to have proper relationships with others, with family members, with the community, with fish and wildlife, and with the Earth. Alaskan elders say that nothing is created outside until it is created or experienced inside first…. In other words, what we do outside through our actions is a reflection of what we do inside to ourselves. We trash the environment outside because we are trashing our own internal environment. We create conflict outside because we are conflicted inside. We criticize and judge others because we are critical and judgmental of ourselves inside.[10]

9 "Whitewashed Hope," Cultural Survival, November 24, 2020. https://www.culturalsurvival.org/news/whitewashed-hope-message-10-indigenous-leaders-and-organizations

10 Ilarion (Larry) Merculieff, "Arctic Traditional Knowledge and Wisdom: Changes in the North American Arctic," CAFF Assessment Series Reporrt NO. 14, April 2017, p. 29 file:///Users/Antonia2016iMac/Desktop/TK_Wisdom_North_American_Arctic_2017.pdf

I have not felt judged in the places we visit around the world; on the contrary, I always feel genuinely welcomed into the cultures we have the privilege to explore. Maybe this is due to hiring local guides who lead with the utmost care for the wildlife, landscape, and people who live on it. We don't arrive as tourists, but as explorers eager to get on the road less traveled for a glimpse of another corner of this magnificent world. We extend the respect and appreciation that goes into the "proper relationship" Larry Merculieff describes, and we receive the same, at the very least, from those we meet.

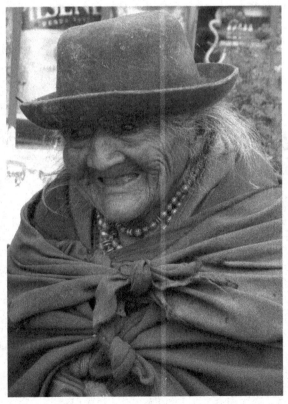

A friendly face in Ecuador. *(Photo: Judy B. Nussenblatt)*

Susan Barron, for example, recalled her amazement at the openness and sincerity of Maasai warriors she met during a trip to Tanzania with her Pencil Promise organization. They brought school supplies to a girls' school in a women's village founded by a group of tribal women dedicated to turning the tide for girls' lives through education. Sitting around a fire in the desert with the male warriors one evening, Susan learned how the girls' education would impact the entire tribe. She asked for permission before taking pictures of them in their striking beaded regalia and painted faces, and as night fell and the conversation got going, the men said they were glad she and her group were there to assist in their girls' education.

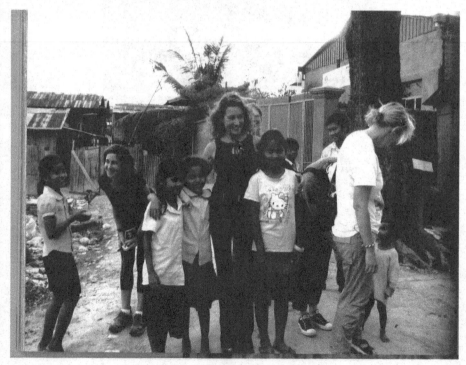

STAT travelers Jen (left), Susan B. (center), and Sam with children in Phnom Penh. *(Photo: Judy B. Nussenblatt)*

"But you know," they told her, "this will make us extinct."

"Extinct—why?" she asked.

"When our sisters get an education they will want to go to town and get a job in an office. They're not going to want to live in a dung hut and wait for us to come home with the herd at the end of the day. We're the last. After us, there will be no more. But this is not a good life for girls. We are happy for these girls to have an education."

After taking that in, as well as the fact that these men were willing to open up to her in the first place, Susan told them she had seen boys in the girls' school and asked why they were there.

"We want the boys to see how smart the girls are," one said.

Susan had quickly let go of any preconceived ideas she may have had about Maasai warriors and relished the chance to hear their views. Her experience reminds me of when I set aside my preconceived notions about men's ability to open up in spiritual rituals during a group trip. A few of my friends were asking for a couples trip, but I resisted the idea because I wasn't sure the men would engage. I also thought they may be harder to lead through the planned agenda of a trip, including morning yoga, the talking stick ceremony, and other activities. On our trips, you don't leave the scene to go off on a run on your own or bow out of something—it's all about the group dynamic.

I had a lot of trepidation, but I knew the couples who would be traveling and threw this venture out there to try something new. Interestingly enough, it really worked. The men got into the ceremonial piece of it and spoke with an open heart. The beauty of a STAT trip is that you come with the itinerary in hand and know the basics of what to expect. You don't have to make decisions, just follow my lead and the instructions of my expert guides. Surprises do show up, but with the exception of our couples' trip to Columbia, they've never been dangerous. On our couples' trek to the Lost City in Columbia, the flash floods that shifted our gears and rugged outdoor sleeping arrangements were not fun. But the men took it in stride, especially since the women were, for the most part, their usual hearty, strong, resilient, and humorous selves, even during sleepless nights hanging in hammocks to keep a safe distance from the creepy crawlies on the ground.

Having the guys there was almost comforting because we were all in this together and we knew they witnessed a new side of us. In the toughest moments, the men looked at us resolutely, as if thinking, *If they can do it, I can do it.* I gladly learned that my assumptions about men being difficult to lead or unwilling to genuinely engage were wrong.

Loosening our hold on assumptions and snap judgments is a natural effect of mindfulness, with its here-and-now attention that eases us away from preconceived ideas and thoughts about the past or future. As it filters from wellness centers to schools and even the business world, mindfulness is a modern take on practices developed in Hinduism and Buddhism thousands of years ago, but who cares where it came from? Focusing on what is present rather than filtering everything through our self-obsessed, "me-first" ego perspective can only do us and our society good.

The nonjudgmental aspect of mindfulness meditation wears away the irrational ideas we build up over the years, and when we stop judging we realize how much those ideas used to drive our behavior. In her book on bringing mindfulness to business leadership, Deborah Rowland describes what sounds a lot like the Aleut people's heal-the-inside-first view. "In my corporate roles it became very clear that I had to be in the right place personally before I could skillfully lead or do anything.... This ability to tune into and regulate the self, within an evolving system, is the number one inner skill in being able to lead change well," she writes. She adds that the magic happens when inner stillness meets the ability to understand the big structure in which everything works. What she calls seeing through a "systemic lens" the Aleut call being in proper relationship with the environment and the Earth—the biggest "system" we have. Rowland teaches that "staying present is the capacity to look on all experience with deep respect for what is,"[11] which means handling a challenging situation by simply agreeing to what is and then exploring the best outcome from that place of stillness.

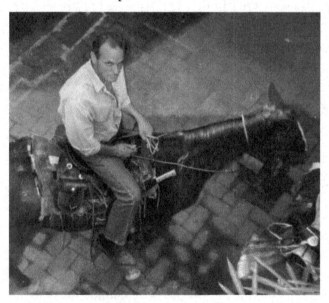

Skip saddled up at his hotel. *(Photo: Author's Archive)*

---

11 Deborah Rowland, *Still Moving: How to Lead Mindful Change*, Wiley, 2017, p. 6.

Staying present with what is gets easier with practice. We naturally face the unknown with a blend of fear and anxiety, even if most of it lies below the surface. But when you get comfortable with your stillness and can access it at will, you can trust yourself to keep steady no matter what comes. You can also trust that your instinct to judge by appearances will fade, leaving room for a calm, clear head. My friend Skip, our adventure travel host in Mexico's Copper Canyon, shared a story with me about finding himself in just that position.

SKIP MCWILLIAMS AND...LET'S CALL HIM "BILLY"

As a business owner until a few years ago in a Mexican region known for drug cartels, particularly the Sinaloa cartel, Skip has a local perspective and personal experience that challenges our typical assumptions. I haven't met a cartel boss myself, but Skip paints a vivid picture that encourages me to toss out a few stereotypes I've picked up over time. Here is Skip's story, as he tells it:

> "The cartels. Aren't you afraid of the danger?" is often thrown at me.

> Reality is so much more interesting than generalities.

> I have a boutique hotel in the green triangle of Mexico.

> It is in the pine forested mountains of Mexico, far from cities and towns. The Sinaloa boys come up from the foothills and hide in the Sierra de Chihuahua.

> Two summers ago, groups of guys with Uzis and assault rifles would occasionally saunter into the dining room of our little hotel, plopping down their assorted armaments

on the tables and chairs. They would politely ask for coffee and pay for some small meal.

This was bad for business, as this screams "cartel" to the tourists whose only knowledge of cartels is in the movies, television and the news media which is also the entertainment business.

Rumor had it that their boss was the second most wanted of the Sinaloa boys in our area. Big shot, apparently. Word also had it that he had one of his houses nearby.

Now I am not a courageous man. But I will jump off a cliff into the water if I am sure the water is deep enough. So I asked around, and as long as anyone could remember this guy was not involved in extortion, kidnapping or anything that had to do with folks not in his industry. In fact, I was told he was expecting me to come calling sooner or later, just the correct neighborly thing to do, I guess.

So one day it was cloudy (we call those tequila days, as there is not much else to do). I went out with a driver until we spotted a car full of Uzis, etc. They were pulled over at a *rancho* having beers and talking. The door was open. The guys had on black vests over black nylon jackets. It looked like they had been wiping their taco-fingers on the lower part of the vests all summer. The guns were grimy except the high surfaces had a burnished patina from constant handling. This was not Hollywood. Guns are always clean in Hollywood.

They apparently knew me and were all smiles and greetings.

"How 'bout I see your boss?"

Some brief walkie-talkie, then, "Follow us."

In a village of ten-by-fifteen-foot adobe two-roomers stands a house right out of Midwest suburbia with a green steel roof. Leading up was a forty-foot-wide cement bridge over a two-foot stream. There was a low wall around the place. He greeted me on the front porch. I introduced myself. He did not. Let's call him Billy.

I was not apprehensive because I knew three things:

First: Billy can see through people easily, or he would not have lived as long as he has.

Second: Men in his position waste no energy on extraneous or capricious action.

Third: If I am honest and open, he will have nothing to fear and no reason to kill me.

As is the tradition of the sierra, I had a bottle of tequila which I placed on the table, "*Nuestro entender está en el fondo de esta botella, y para encontrarlo hay que vaciarla.* Our understanding is in the bottom of this bottle, and to find it we must empty the bottle."

Glasses appeared.

This is vertical country. When someone draws me a map, it is not left and right, north and south like a world seen from above.... *It is a side view of the ups and downs that you need to do to get somewhere.* Horses here are born on slopes so steep you can't walk them. Horses from elsewhere are injured beyond repair the first day here. Billy was born here. He was about between forty-five and fifty, over six feet I think, not skinny or wiry, not fat but solid muscle. He can easily disappear into the pine slopes within seconds and keep going a long way.

He asked why I had been gone from the sierra and when I started explaining about the health of a family member, he waved off the explanation as unnecessary. He spoke of Gringos and halted himself to ask if the term was insulting. We agreed that our employees were essential to our businesses and we would be nothing without them. And vice versa. We talked about the fine points of people and organizational management. I have never met a CEO of a good-sized company who had anything surpassing his insights on the dynamics of people functioning in organizations.

He was trying to start a sawmill for the community, but he was blocked by the corruption of the timber business with cutting permits handed out as political favors. He mentioned that he would have to 'clean there' somewhere down the road, so the timber could flow to the community sawmill. I did not ask him to elaborate.

He had several walkie talkies on the table that needed attention every minute or so. Reports from *halcones*, falcons, watchers in high places reporting who was on the single road that passes through that part of the sierra. He was fully aware of all dimensions, human and otherwise, of his 360 degrees. He lives on constant adrenalin, ready and very capable at every moment of springing to kill or disappear. It seemed his first priority was to survive till nightfall.

He was interested in our conversation because it was business, and the discussion was to know who he was dealing with. I explained that his guys showing up was bad for the business which is the principal employer of the area. He was born in the community and his neighbors, including many years ago his own mother, worked at the hotel cleaning rooms. He said not to worry.

"Now," he said, "I want you to give me money just one time, one time only."

I explained that I had several thousand dollars cash on me, which I intended for a community project. I asked him what he wanted me to do with it, give it to him or the people. He did not hesitate *"para la gente.* For the people."

His concern for his community was real. His insights as a businessman were the stuff of advanced management seminars. I was in the presence of a sophisticated manager. Brilliant in business. Brilliant in survival. Why is he not running a major corporation? It is because he is a mestizo in a part of the country where the mix is with the Rarámuri, considered primitive by the economically dominant Mexican culture. With no chance of more than a sixth-grade education, and his bloodline, he would be lucky to land a job as a baggage handler at an airport in the city.

It is said that a human being is happiest when they can utilize their abilities. In the sierra are many men of ability to whom Mexican society is closed. So partly out of need to manifest their abilities, partly out of resentment, many chose green industries not accepted by society. How ironic that dope stocks are now very hot on Wall Street. They are still excluded. So they choose to operate outside of accepted society.

Later, I asked my manager about Billy, because he was nothing like the picture in my mind of "The Cartel." I even wondered to myself if Billy was really number two in the Cartel like the newspapers said.

When I asked about Billy, my manager fell silent. Then in almost a whisper, he told me this story:

"Billy saved my life. Praise God. I owe him the life I have now. I was lost until he and Jesus saved me. You know I am a missionary for Jesus all because of Billy. Praise the name of the Lord. I had fallen for many years into sin. I drank, had many women, abused my wife, and neglected her and the children. I was the worst. I have Billy and the Lord to thank for my salvation. I am now six years sober, a good husband and father. I follow the lord. Praise Him. Billy is a great man. I was horrible and did not deserve to live. Billy is the *compadre* of the brother of my wife. My brother-in-law had enough of how I treated his sister which was really the work of the devil in me. He asked his *compadre* Billy to have me killed. I was summoned and a friend took me to see Billy. There was me, my friend and two other guys who I did not know. Billy told us he was going to kill the three of us. My friend interceded on my behalf and after much talk, convinced Billy not to kill me. The experience literally scared me onto the right road and to Jesus. Praise God."

I had to ask, "Why were you so scared? Well, he let you off. How do you know he was really serious about killing you? Seems like a pretty nice guy."

"He made me dispose of the other two bodies."

Reality is so much more interesting than generalities.

No cute lizards or mountain rabbits in that story, but it brings home the point. Not even a drug cartel boss is as one-dimensional as the media and film industry would have us believe. Our own encounters with the unknown will probably be a lot milder, such as losing battery power on a flashlight helmet while bicycling in the dark. But being fully present, with heart and mind open and humble, is a good way to let situations weave themselves into our lives in the best way for all involved.

ନ୍ତ

FOR REFLECTION

1. Recall at least two people you formed an opinion about when you first met and then later realized you had completely "read them wrong."

2. What kind of general assumptions do you make, or used to make, about the opposite sex? How have specific men or women proved your assumptions false?

3. Consider a difficult/challenging experience that comes up frequently for you (not an abusive situation, which needs your action to keep you physically safe). Close your eyes and imag-

ine you are facing the difficult moment (getting a phone call from someone who triggers you, having a migraine, opening a bill, facing down an impending deadline, etc.). Instead of pushing back with frustration, sadness, or anger, simply say to yourself, "This is what it is, and I am calm." Relax your jaw and shoulders and focus on your breath. Keep relaxing in the stillness. The next time you face the experience in real life, try to do the same. Keep note of what ideas or guidance come to you in the stillness.

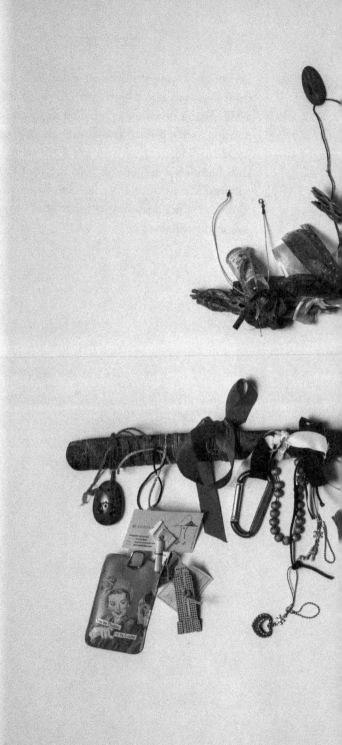

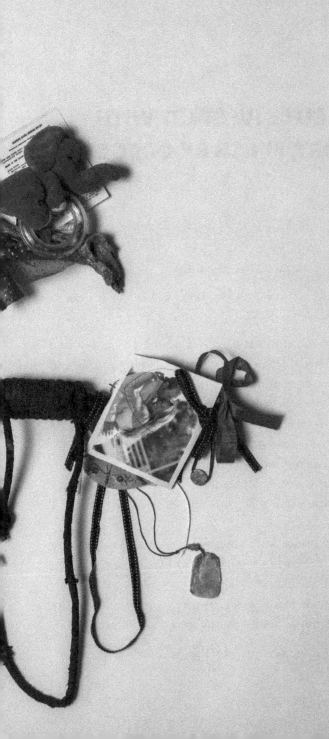

CHAPTER 7

PRINCIPLE IV: START WITH EFFORT, FINISH BY GRACE

Trust. Wait. Let go.
We are being led.
We are being guided.

—MELODY BEATTIE[1]

WHEN I ARRANGE AN ADVENTURE travel journey, I do my best to cover all the details, from hiring expert trekking guides and locals who can introduce us to the culture to organizing the crazy variety of transportation we usually need to get from A to B in off-the-beaten path locations. I consider these plans, which take months, to be 80 percent of what makes a trip work. I leave the other 20 percent to God, the higher power, or the universe, whatever you'd like to call it. In terms of the unexpected help or all-around-good resolution that pops up just when we need it, I call it *the magic*.

I've learned to always leave something open in an adventure trip itinerary and, as best I can, in every day I walk the earth. You have to leave room for magic.

Another word for this is grace. When we are unexpectedly helped in body, mind, or soul—through no effort of our own—

---

1   Melody Beattie, *The Language of Letting Go.* Hazelden, 2009, p. x.

we call it an act of grace. These experiences leave us awestruck, humbled, and mystified in the face of proof that there's more going on in our lives than meets the eye. As grace falls on us time after time over the years, it gets easier to trust that things will work out for the best, and we can relax and be open to what comes rather than constantly try to control everything. I found myself releasing into this trust one day in Cambodia when two of my girls got lost during a long hike through the jungle. We were a large group that year, thirteen women, and the day started with exploring a village. We meandered in pairs and small groups, taking our time to stop in front of shops to admire handmade jewelry, water bottles wrapped in handwoven covers, and ready-to-drink fresh coconuts with straws. At midmorning we finally filed in behind our two guides to start our day-long trek through the dense timber and bamboo. I couldn't see those at the very back, but I knew Judy would be the last among them, as she always stayed behind to take pictures. I also assumed that one guide would remain in the back to stay with the slower hikers, leaving the other guide up front to keep track of the rest. I arranged the guides this way so I could always rest assured that everyone would have a guide nearby. Little did I know that Judy and Susan B. were still in the village and had not seen us leave.

The two stragglers were hunkered down with their cameras in the main shopping area watching a couple of roosters go at each other in an impromptu cock fight. A little crowd gathered as the dust and feathers flew, giving Judy and Susan more action to capture. After the roosters got it out of their system and strutted away, the girls wiped themselves off, looked up, and noticed that no one in our group was around. They walked through the entire village again to look for us, and with no luck, decided to start on the trail on their own. About twenty minutes in they came to a fork in the road and had no idea which way we had gone.

Heading to the left, they walked for another ten minutes without hearing any calls, laughter, or other signs of humans up ahead, so they headed back to the village. Chewing on power bars they'd stuffed in their backpacks, they settled in to wait for us, figuring we'd eventually realize they were missing and come looking.

Two hours later, our group stopped at a platform by a waterfall where the guides started to prepare lunch. I made a quick head count and discovered we were missing two, and as I stared at the trail, willing Judy and Susan to appear, I silently scolded myself for not making sure one of the guides had stayed at the back. I would never make that mistake again. Brooke, who was a daily runner in great shape, volunteered to run back to find them. She ran the entire length of the trail that had taken us almost three-and-a-half hours to walk and found the two lost souls in the village, relaxing under a tree. *La di da*... They weren't even freaked out.

While Brooke was running to the rescue, I had a moment of nerve-racking anxiety. We were in a foreign land. Anything could have happened out there...but my gut told me they were okay, and I trusted we would all be together soon, and safe. I was smack dab in the 20 percent realm, the zone of no control. I had done all I could, including hiring two guides who, as it turned out, knew how to contact someone who could get a vehicle to that village and bring those girls to the end of the trail by the time we got there. The magic of all this came to me in retrospect while talking to the girls about that day. We realized we'd dodged a bullet by leaving from that village rather than being dropped off at a remote trailhead somewhere in the jungle. Judy and Susan easily retraced their path back to the village that was, by then, very familiar to them, and they felt safe. So they spent a few more hours there than planned—so what? They enjoyed each other's company and got a much deeper sense of the vibe and community in that village than the rest of us. They trusted that all was well, and because it was, we could joke about it later—Geez, remember that first hike? We almost lost you guys!

When the trust sinks in, it's very freeing. You take a breath in your heart, relax, and open to the magic.

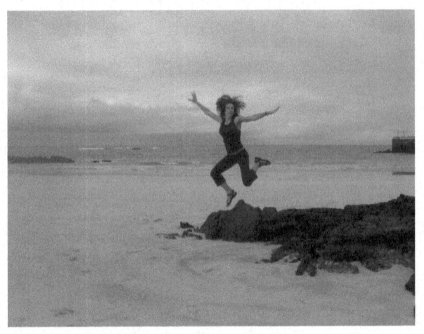

Fleet-of-foot Brooke. *(Photo: Judy B. Nussenblatt)*

GRACE BY ANY OTHER NAME

American spiritual teacher Adyashanti, whose path began with years of study and practice in Zen, describes grace through that Buddhist lens. To him, grace is the essence of our being, the "vast space of peace, of stillness, of ultimate wellbeing"[2] that we share

---

2 Adyashanti, *Falling Into Grace: Insights on the End of Suffering.* Sounds True, 2011, p. 230.

with everything else in the universe. He writes that stepping away from our ego self and inviting the divine to take over opens us to grace:

> We have to let go of the illusion that we are in control of our life. When we hand it over, we'll find ourselves falling into grace, falling into this clarity and openness and love, falling right into the grace of awakening from separation, where we realize our true spiritual essence: this beautiful, unknown, unborn presence which manifests as everything we see.[3]

Adyashanti's view of grace as the state in which we know we're connected to everything reminds me of the spirituality of the Kaqchikel Maya, the Indigenous people we learned about and met on our unforgettable trip to Guatemala in 2018.

The cultural and geographic diversity in this small country is mind-boggling—it's home to everything from ancient Mayan temples and Spanish colonial cities to rain forests and vibrant Caribbean towns, not to mention three spewing active volcanoes. But evidently, as we learned, what truly makes this country unique are the Maya, whose distinctive culture and centuries-old traditions continue to thrive today. We made the steep four-mile hike up the forested side of the Pacaya volcano as it belched smoke, and at the top a shaman performed a Mayan blessing ceremony for us, which was pure magic.

The air had been calm on our way up, but when we reached the top a blustery wind whipped through our hair. We wandered around the top of the volcano for a while, thrilling to the view of mountains all around us, some with fine tips that looked like carved pyramids. The shaman who soon joined us wore a

---

3   Ibid., p. 226.

red ceremonial headscarf and multicolored bead necklaces. He got on his knees and drew a white circle on the dark volcanic ground with some kind of powder. Inside the circle he prepared a small fire using green, orange, blue, brown, and red candlesticks carefully gathered into a raised starburst pattern with the wicks in the center. After lighting the candles, he swept up his hands, as if inviting the fire to climb upward. As he chanted, our guide explained that he was praying to ask the spirits of the ancestors for permission to hold this ceremony. He then gestured for us to hold hands and form a circle around the small fire. He continued to chant in his ancient language, and although we did not understand the words, we felt the sacred bond that connected us to him and this extraordinary place. Our guides translated the words he spoke to each of us individually as he blessed us with fragrant smoke of sage. We repeated those chants as he smudged us head to toe, first along the front and, when we turned around, the back.

As I stood in the circle with our intimate group, the gusts of wind felt like the ancestor spirits dancing around us. Years later, as I was reminiscing about that ceremony with my friend Joy, she recalled the gratitude we all felt for being able to experience this place with this spiritual man:

> He invited us to offer up something, a message we hoped would reach a higher being. After he blessed us one by one, we leaned in with a little bow to acknowledge the gift. Everyone felt grateful for the blessing and the beautiful opportunity to share the energy of someone like him. I believe he felt our deep unity as a group as he blessed us with good health and overall good fortune.

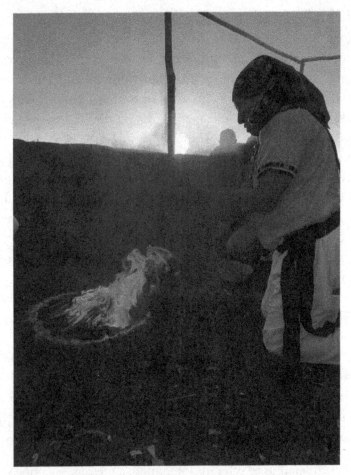

A shaman prepares a ritual fire for our blessing ceremony on Pacaya
mountain in Guatemala. *(Photo: Author's Archive)*

We learned that *utzilaj,* *laslrm,* and *winakirem* are Mayan
words to describe goodness, life, and our relationship to the
universe. The Mayan way of life is all about that relationship.
As anthropologists put it, to the Maya, God is a unified cosmic
force and "the cosmic order is one of perfect harmony and balance between natural and metaphysical [spirit world] forces....

It is seen as the duty of (Maya) humans to approximate cosmic harmony on earth."[4] It's not surprising, then, that the Maya are such strong activists for conserving Guatemala's forests, rivers, and wildlife. I am inspired by that and by the reverence they bring to their lives through rituals and careful attention to keeping the natural balance in their bodies and the environment.

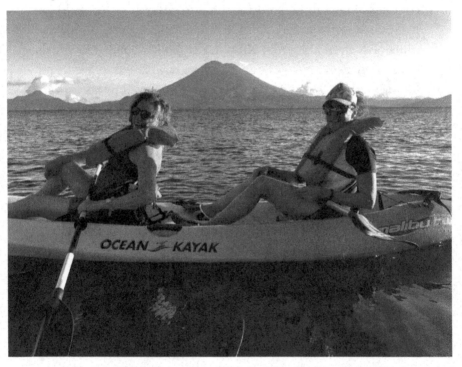

Blissed-out STAT kayakers on Guatemala's Lake Atitlán, one of the most beautiful lakes in the world. Surrounded by volcanoes, the basin formed when a volcano erupted and collapsed about eighty-four thousand years ago. *(Photo: Author's Archive)*

---

4   Robert M. Hill II & Edward F. Fischer, "An Ethnohistorical Approach to Kaqchikel Maya Ethnopsychology," *Ancient Mesoamerica*, vol. 10 (1999), p. 317.

We can think of grace as a sort of divine intervention, or as a state of perfect connection as described by Adyashanti and as honored by the Maya. Other meanings of grace come from religion, such as the Jewish outlook that God is merciful in spite of our not measuring up to that mercy. We're taught that even if we don't rack up a lot of good deeds, God will forgive our short-comings. This can be hard for some to believe, as Rabbi Elliot J. Cosgrove of the Park Avenue Synagogue in New York City explained. Even after Yom Kippur, the Jewish holiday in which God forgives and purifies us because we have fasted, prayed, and forgiven and made amends to others, we still need to ask for forgiveness. One reason, he says, is that "although God has accepted our atonement, we harbor doubt as to whether God has in fact forgiven us." The sin is "doubting God's grace."[5]

Christianity has a different take on grace with the belief that since people are born as sinners—including the sin of being separated from God—their only hope is to be healed by God's grace. Not all Christians believe in "original sin," though, and some are more "Eastern wisdom" leaning than others. Serene Jones, for example, the president of Union Theological Seminary in New York City, defines grace as God's permanent presence in us and in "all existence." She believes that God is a mystery, the loving divine reality of the universe beyond our imagining.[6]

We use the word grace for more down-to-earth experiences too, such as staying in someone's good graces, saying grace before a meal, accepting defeat or advice with grace, addressing certain royalty as "your grace," or describing a typically disagreeable person's saving grace of a sense of humor. In music there's the little

---

5   Elliot J. Cosgrove, Sermon: "After the Fast," September 18, 2021, https://pasyn. org/sermon/after-fast

6   Serene Jones, *Call It Grace: Finding Meaning in a Fractured World.* Viking, 2019, pp. xvi, xviii, p. 3.

flip of a grace note, and in Greek mythology we have the three Graces, the sister goddesses who bestow beauty, charm, and creativity. This is the meaning of grace that, along with the sudden gift of magic, comes closest to my principle of starting with effort and finishing by grace.

Trekking life with grace means having a life purpose that includes being your best self for your own sake and for others. You take care of yourself to live life to the fullest, because life is a gift, and only by being your best self can you give the most. If more people think about their life in terms of having a purpose that makes the world a better place, even the smallest corner of the world, rather than merely "a career," we may have a better dialogue about all the challenges we face. Early on when I was searching for a purpose, I took time to follow the clues that crossed my path by little acts of grace: an invitation to a vision quest in Colorado, unexpected advice and help from a new STAT traveler on her way to becoming a hugely successful entrepreneur. With my mission in place, the gifts kept coming, like finding philanthropy expert Lydia to help me bring a game-changing new element to our trips.

When you make the effort to find your mission, you set the magic in motion. It doesn't have to be a grand mission to end global poverty or find a cure for cancer (although that would be nice)—a mission can mean *being a good person* in ways that are right in front of you: being the one who always helps the neighbors, no questions asked, bringing in the mail if they're elderly and shoveling the sidewalk for the whole block. A mission can mean being a great mother or a friend people can really count on. A mission can be working in your chosen career with a generous, loving attitude that makes it a nourishing place for everyone. To live like this is to walk with grace and dignity.

As a mom, I always said, first and foremost, that all I ever wanted for my two boys was for them to be good. Everything else follows. As long as they had a stable starting point early on, such as what they learned while studying for their bar mitzvahs that came at age thirteen, I believed they would be good. And they are. A mentor helped me nurture this idea during my formative years as a young mother. Jewish theologian and radio talk show host Dennis Prager had recorded a series of tapes called "Dennis Teaches the Torah," his lessons and reflections on the first five books of the Old Testament. As I listened to these tapes on my daily walks, I learned about Jewish philosophy and took to heart the ideas Prager frequently shared about bringing up kids. One of his recent online commentaries harkens back to his messages from those tapes. If we ask a child, "What do you want to be?" most will name a profession like "a doctor," "a teacher, "a pilot," or "a firefighter," he writes. If we tell our child to answer, "I want to be a good person," that conversation could change a "child's life—and the world—for the better," because, as a rule,

> people become what they want to become. If you devote the entire first half of your life, including your most formative years, to being a good student in order to be a good professional, you probably will become...a good student and a good professional.... The moment you tell your child to answer, "a good person" you will have to start communicating that you value their character more than their grades.[7]

---

7 Dennis Prager, "Growing Up to Be Good Is More Important Than Career," *The Daily Signal,* October 1, 2019, https://www.dailysignal.com/2019/10/01/growing-up-to-be-good-is-more-important-than-career/

This was inspiring to me because it resonated with my own quest to be purposeful and seek out a deeper meaning in life than just a career or profession can bring. I wasn't religious in the traditional sense, but studying the Torah in this simple, ritual way gave me a foundation of understanding about what matters most. Over the years, those priorities have naturally blended into everything I do.

In my mission to encourage women to be their best selves, I set up travels that challenge us to be more in our bodies and open up to honest reflection and connection. I also make sure we'll have a damn good time along the way. Even when I visit with friends over dinner or a walk, this is what we talk about—how to be our best selves, how to walk our talk and do the right thing. As Gina would say, "Sharing is caring."

The magic of grace can appear at any time to offer up an idea or solution or, in a tense situation, strike like a lightning bolt to erase the anxiety. This happened to me recently when I was on vacation with Paul in France. On the third day of our trip, I got an email saying that the domain name for my business website had disappeared. The site was gone, missing, nowhere—when I typed in the address on my phone's browser, I came up with a blank page, bupkis. All my emails were diverted back to sender as "unknown addressee." How could my entire website and business email disappear in a snap? Panic set in as my amazingly smart website guys back in New York said they needed tons of information to give to the hosting company so they could fix their error. Crack open the security? Potentially lose the site that held decades of blog posts and business emails? What a nightmare. After a few days of this, Paul stepped in to remind me who I was. "Erin, you always say, trust the universe. You've got to step back and take a couple of deep breaths." Paul likes to chide me a lot, in a loving way, about 'trusting in the universe,' but this day he sincerely meant it, and it worked. I let go and my shoulders dropped as if they'd been hanging by two wires. I took a breath and calm rushed in. All my anxiety melted away, just like that.

For the next three days as my web guys did their thing, I trusted everything would get resolved. And it did. The hosting company found the glitch and sent their apologies, promising it would never happen again. But what if things hadn't gone that way, and there was no fix? The worst case scenario would be losing decades of information, images, and data, but would that really be so bad? Websites can be rebuilt. Email addresses can be collected again. New pictures can be taken. I could just start over. It's actually comforting to know that no matter what, I can move on, reset, and start again. Relaxing into this is letting go and inviting grace.

The story of the book you're holding also starts with a jolt of the magic we call grace. In 2019 I was thinking about writing something about STAT and our adventures, but it was just that, a thought. One day I went to a friend's house to pick her up for a hike, and she asked if I would mind if a friend of hers joined us. I ended up spending most of the hike alongside her friend who hiked at my pace while my friend followed a bit more slowly. I mentioned to the woman that I was thinking about writing a book and trying to organize my thoughts, and she said her husband was a writer who specialized in helping others do just that—tell their stories. I got his information and met with him, and although it didn't seem like a fit, talking to him encouraged me to seriously look for someone who could coach me and get me started. Talking to that new acquaintance's husband made my idea about the book more real, and sure enough, doors opened, people appeared with suggestions, and I found the assistance I needed to get things rolling. Meeting that quick-paced hiker was no accident or mere coincidence. It was one more uncanny, out-of-the-blue, amazing act of grace.

CR

FOR REFLECTION

1. What is your life purpose or mission?

2. When you think of grace, which meaning among the many described in this chapter first comes to mind? Who shares this understanding of grace with you?

3. Recall a positive experience that came to you as a complete surprise, a magical gift. What problem did this "act of grace" solve or what other impact did it have on your life?

4. Think of a time or two when you responded gracefully to a difficult or uncomfortable situation. How did it feel, and how did others respond to you?

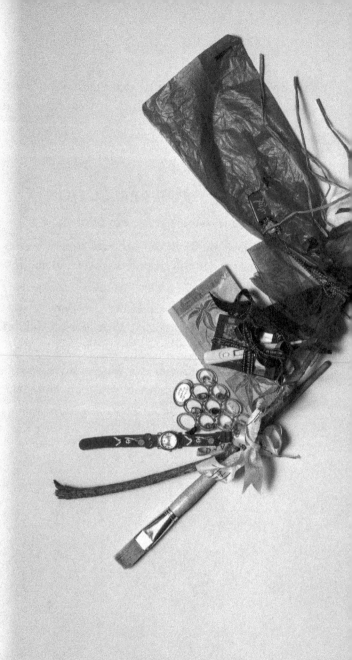

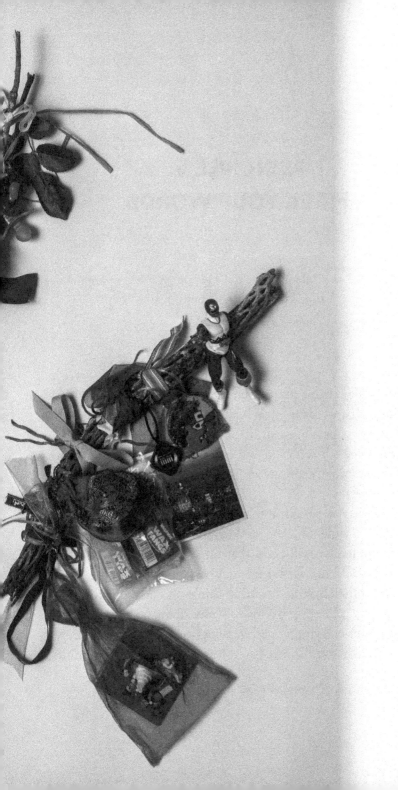

CHAPTER 8

PRINCIPLE V: MARK YOUR WORDS

Intention is a force in nature,
like gravity, but more powerful.

—DEEPAK CHOPRA[1]

ONE OF THE SIMPLEST WAYS I've found to trek life with grace is to start the day with a positive intention. When I go through my morning ritual of setting my intention to navigate through my day as the best person I can be, no matter what may come, the intention sticks. It settles in and guides me in the small and big things. We create intentions with words, either as thoughts or by writing or reading.

The earlier we set our intention, preferably before we get out of bed or as a ritual of some kind before we do anything else, the more grounded we will be in that intention. For me, the ritual sinks in most deeply when I meditate on my power words before doing any other routine morning things like making coffee or checking my phone and email. Now, doing anything before making coffee is saying something, because everyone who knows me knows how much I love my coffee ritual. Those ten minutes

---

1   Deepak Chopra, *The Spontaneous Fulfillment of Desire.* Harmony Books, 2003, p. 208.

spent pouring hot water into my Chemex, inhaling the aroma of my favorite locally roasted coffee as the water gently soaks in... Those are precious moments for me. But they are my reward for first conscientiously setting my intention to walk the earth with a good heart.

WORDS, INTENTIONS, AND RITUAL

Over the years I have accumulated a set of power words, adding them to my repertoire one by one until one day they became "my words." Because there are eight words, I aligned them with the seven chakras, the energy centers of the body, and one additional chakra I imagined hovering about six inches above my head for the last word, "love." Their meaning and resonance are such a part of me that I had them engraved into a necklace—some people like dangling their initials or birthstone on a chain; I like my power words. As I sit in front of Ganesha in the morning, I spend twenty minutes breathing in these words to fill myself with their essence. I begin with the word that embraces the first chakra in the lowest level of the body and work my way up:

Clarity: Clearly seeing and understanding life as it is and what it can be. An experience I had many years ago always comes to mind when I meditate on this word. Out of the blue, my thinking became foggy; things just didn't connect right away. I would ask myself, wouldn't it be nice if I had a windshield wiper in my brain to erase this fogginess? This was the metaphor I kept imagining as I prayed for the condition to go away. I finally went to the doctor, who gave me a blood test and found I had a high mercury count. This may have built up from the mercury fillings in my teeth and from eating a lot of foods high in mercury, like tuna, every day. I replaced those fillings, changed my diet, took some functional medicine supplements with spirulina and seaweed to counteract the mercury in my system, and gradually my clarity returned.

Consciousness: Subjective awareness or, according to some, just awareness itself. As Sam Harris teaches, we may be conscious of things going on around us thanks to what our senses allow us to taste, hear, see, touch, and smell, but the big story is about consciousness, our internal awareness. We meditate, he says, to let go of the belief that there is a separate "me" looking out at the world through our eyes. Instead, we can experience awareness/consciousness directly. He calls this the *intrinsic selflessness of consciousness*. In meditation we can move beyond the mind.

Equilibrium: A state of balance. My equilibrium comes about in my rituals around exercise. I need to move my body every day, whether it be walking, hiking, biking, skiing, yoga, weight training, or Pilates. My emotional and physical stance, my presence in the world as a whole-body human being, comes from my relationship with my body. This keeps my equilibrium victorious.

Effort. Doing, attempting, taking action. I say "trust in the universe," but that doesn't mean relinquishing effort. Effort should not be taken lightly. The universe is not going to rain down the fulfillment of your dreams if you don't make the effort. Effort is key in life; you have to make an effort to be a good friend, a good wife, a good mother, to plan a trip, to eat healthy, to exercise right, to keep your sanity, to be compassionate. You have to make an effort in everything you do. This is not a dry run, not a coasting through life, not a free-for-all—we need to make intentional efforts every day. I respect, honor, and encourage people to make tremendous efforts in life. Sometimes we reap the benefits and sometimes we don't, or at least we don't think we do. Trekking with grace means finding the gift in every outcome.

Grace: Something that just comes, in ways you may never have dreamed. Effort comes from the bottom of your feet to the top of your head, and grace comes from the top of your head down to the bottom of your feet. That's why effort and grace always go together—they're kissing cousins. Even the smallest effort, such as feeling vulnerable and admitting defeat or power-lessness, can be enough to be open yourself to acts of grace.

Intention: An aim that comes from the heart, the intended way you want to live your life. Living should be intentional, as I tell my girls when I ask them to bring a symbol of the intention they care about most at this moment in their life to put on the talking stick. In this sense of the word, an intention is not a set goal, but an openness to flow with the truth as it comes along. If you're at the top of the ladder in your profession at fifty, you don't quit intending how to live, you keep going. As a human being, you keep moving up. As the River Clarion says in Mary Oliver's poem, "Imagine everything you can imagine, then keep on going."[2]

Integrity: The quality of doing the right thing. I believe integrity is the number-one characteristic of a good person. We say that something built well has "structural integrity," and we see this in people who develop their hearts, minds, and actions around a moral compass and genuine care for others and the world.

Love: The word for the universal understanding of the emotion/force we feel for ourselves, others, and all that is. Love connects us to our friends, family, neighbors, community, and world at large. Love has the last say. It's no cliché that all you need is love.

As I sit in meditation, I pull up each word through the center of my body and feel their energy light up my chakras. In my

---

2   Mary Oliver, "At the River Clarion," in *Devotions: The Selected Poems of Mary Oliver*. Penguin, 2017, p. 86.

mind's eye, these energy centers become more radiant, sending vibrant life into every cell. When I get to the eighth chakra that spins above my head, the power word "love" becomes an intense physical feeling that pours down into me. I am immersed in calm and happiness.

Some mornings I meditate with other words, such as my TM mantra or a guided audio from Sam Harris, Joe Dispenza, or Tara Brach. And sometimes I choose a breathing practice or simply stay with the silence. It depends on what is happening in my life, what I need to sit with. These variations come and go, but one thing never changes—making time to do it. Self-discipline can sound like putting pressure on yourself, but it's just the opposite. Keeping a regular practice that improves your life at the deepest level is an expression of love. It is love in action, making you more fit to be the best person you can be wherever today's path takes you.

On my adventure journeys, I use rituals like morning yoga and the talking stick ceremony to help women connect with their inner selves. Yoga and outdoor sports bring us closer to understanding how our bodies work, from our muscles to our internal organs, and our physical selves have as much to tell us as our minds and souls. My trips are retreats, journeys of self-exploration that send a woman home a better person. There's a shift in one's being. Some notice it right away, and others maybe weeks or months after they get back, but there is always a shift because they return restored. Yoga in particular is a restorative practice. I include it as an internal practice for a shift in their psyche, their soul, their personal being.

When you're in a yoga class you're practicing with other people, so you feel like a warrior, but in fact you're practicing for your own internal release. It manifests differently with everyone—stiff people have a hard time with a lot of the poses because they have boundaries and have to learn how to live within them. Very flexible people like myself have to learn how to get boundaries. My body can go beyond the poses, and that's not good either. So there is a happy medium to find, and practice is the journey to discovering the equilibrium that you and your body seek.

SHAMANS AND RITUAL

Words have been connected to healing since ancient times in every culture. According to my childhood picture book of mythology, the ancient Greeks gave Apollo the double role of god of medicine and poetry, pairing up the two arts. In Kabbalah, or Jewish mysticism, each letter of the Hebrew alphabet is said to contain power and a life of its own, and learning the symbolism of the letters is a pathway to spiritual enlightenment and gifts such as the power to heal. I first learned about this symbolism when I began studying Kabbalah at age forty, when my sons were studying for their bar mitzvahs. The timing was an interesting coincidence because Jewish law traditionally allowed women to start reading the Bible and studying the Torah at age forty. I studied with Eliyahu Jian, a New York-based spiritual teacher who had a way of making Kabbalah a down-to-earth path for everyday life. One big takeaway from his lessons was that we should take responsibility for everything we do—there are no victims. We're not perfect and we can transform and evolve from our mistakes. As another Kabbalah teacher at New York's Kabbalah Centre once said, *We all make mistakes, and that's why God puts erasers on pencils.* Our mistakes are gifts that help us become better versions of ourselves.

Another major lesson from Eliyahu was that we should not let negative thoughts take over when conflicts come along, but instead use positive thoughts to be proactive and find solutions. The wisdom of Kabbalah teaches us to pay attention to whether our thoughts are negative or positive, acknowledge them, and then be positive and proactive instead of reactive. By the time COVID-19 came along, I was accustomed to looking at my thoughts in this way and to choosing the proactive approach. Instead of thinking adventure travel was over for me because it would take too long for things to open up again, I rolled up my sleeves and planned a trip to Bolivia for May 2021. This gave the girls who signed up something to look forward to— we penciled it in and when it looked like that spring wouldn't work, erased it and planned for November 2021 instead. The pandemic was still too rampant at that time, so we rescheduled it again for November 2022. No one asked for their deposit back because they were all thinking positive. Instead of spinning down a negative spiral of naysaying or fear about long-term COVID, we were being proactive about planning more body-and-soul-nurturing retreats.

Kabbalah is a fascinating exploration of words and symbols that has opened new doors of understanding for me alongside other wisdom traditions. To this day, for example, Native American medicine men and shamans throughout the world draw on ancient traditions to chant and drum in their healing rituals. Using words for their rhythm and meaning and combining them with drumming draws the shaman into an altered state of consciousness where he or she can communicate with the spirit world to bring healing to the "patient." In her book *Kindling the Native Spirit*, Denise Linn, a member of the Cherokee Nation, shares details about drumming's impact on the brain:

> Research has shown that the shamanic beat used around the world, which is about 210 to 220 beats per min-

ute, can catapult your brain waves into a low alpha and theta range. This type of brain activity is associated with heightened senses, creativity, and vivid imagery. When one is in this altered state, it's easier to travel from the physical world into the spiritual realms.[3]

Shamans we've encountered in ceremonies on our trips have tried different ways of jolting us out of ordinary consciousness for a glimpse into another world. During a spirit cleansing ritual in Ecuador's Cochasquí, a mystical land of pyramids and burial mounds dating back to 700 AD, a *yachak*, or shaman, crouched down in front of each of us and blew tobacco smoke into our nostrils with one sharp, powerful snort through a small wooden tube. On that chilly, misty morning, he then fanned us with long condor feathers as we sat around his small ceremonial fire. Eyes closed, we accepted the blessings that heightened our senses and swept us into the mystery of that enchanting place. The shaman's ritual invited us to meld with the sacred intentions of the first people who sat on these highlands to stare at the sky and, with their pyramids, calculate the solstices through the movement of the stars. Beneath the same sky, I felt connected to them as the yachak leaned close, put his hand on top of my head, and blew fragrant tobacco smoke into my third eye.

Traveling to power centers around the world where shamans have been practicing their rituals for thousands of years has been a gift, a blessing that combines adventure and transformation. But we don't have to travel to faraway countries to have these experiences. Here in New York City, I have been working with an urban shaman for almost thirty years. Aleta St. James has a thriving practice as an energy healer and life coach, using her

---

3   Denise Linn, *Kindling the Native Spirit: Sacred Practices for Everyday Life*. Hay House, 2015, p. 87.

natural gifts as a psychic and healer along with the techniques she gathered from years of studying Eastern and Western philosophies, spirituality, rituals, and healing practices. She has traveled all over the world to work with clients, but at the time I met her, she was also traveling on a personal mission to work with Indigenous shamans.

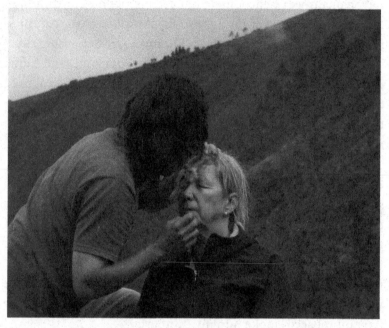

In Ecuador's Cochasquí, the shaman blows smoke into Susan K.'s third eye. *(Photo: Judy B. Nussenblatt)*

Aleta's deepest desire was to have children—twins, in fact— and in places like Peru she sought help to clear the physical, mental, and emotional blocks that had kept her dream at bay. She shared with me that in Peru, a power place where Amazonian shamans have passed on their practices from generation to generation for at least three thousand years, she took part in their rituals and learned how they transferred themselves and others into higher energy fields. "Some do it with drugs," she said, referring to the hallucinogenic substances for which Amazonian shamans are known, "but I do it without drugs. I hold no judgement either way; that's just not my way."

Aleta was determined to use the methods that dramatically shifted the lives of her clients on herself, no matter how long it took or how far she had to travel for the experiences that would heal her issues at the deepest level. She had helped many hard-driven, soul-weary New Yorkers and others rediscover their dreams and achieve them, including women with fertility issues. Word was, "If you stay with Aleta long enough, you'll have your baby." Now it was her turn.

One year in the course of this journey, Aleta joined me and a small group of women on a STAT trip to Wyoming. We were already friends, as I had been seeing her for shamanic healing sessions about four times a year. In Wyoming we learned we also made great travel companions, partly because, according to Aleta, we're both Scorpios: "Scorpio is a sign of transformation," she said. "Like Phoenix rising from the ashes, we take negatives and transform them into positives. It's all about evolution." So far, Aleta's evolution had included moving on from one life calling as a musical theatre actress to another as a psychic, healer, and life coach. Needless to say, I was excited about having her with us in the Wyoming wilderness.

For the talking stick ceremony, Aleta brought an item that symbolized her intention to get pregnant. She was a year or two into her quest, and she recalled that the trip took place during a particularly difficult time:

> I had just had a miscarriage. I was about fifty-one or fif-ty-two at the time and kind of feeling down and won-dering what my next steps were. Erin had said, 'Why

don't you come on my trip?' so I did. It was a magical
trip because even though I know how to change energy,
sometimes you have to go to power points and be with
a group of people to focus in on what you want to manifest in an energy vortex. When we did the circle and
people were talking about what they wanted to manifest,
I talked about wanting twins. I brought a leather pouch
and a simulation of a womb, and I put that in the pouch
and tied it on the stick. As the stick went around I was
visualizing and using all the energy in that place, which
was very strong. I used my own techniques along with
Erin's, but the experience was definitely a catalyst for not
feeling so devastated about the miscarriage.

After the trip, Aleta continued nurturing her intention as she
worked with her clients, and five years later she made headlines
around the world as the oldest American woman to give birth to
twins. Three days before her fifty-seventh birthday, she brought
Francesca and Gian into the world after a successful invitro process. Today, at seventy-five, she is as vibrant and energetic as ever,
raising two teenagers while immersed in her healing practice.

In 2021, I had a session with Aleta to help me deal with the
loss of my dog, Sydney. As I walked up to her fifth-floor studio
on the West Side (there's an elevator, but I still love taking the
stairs like I did back in the day with Cheryl), I knew the next
hour would carry me to a better place. As usual, stepping into
Aleta's inner sanctum was like entering a feminine sanctuary. The
light walls, framed pictures of female gurus and saints, white cov-
erlet on the bed where I would relax against soft white pillows,
and sunlight streaming in felt like a loving maternal embrace.
Aleta sat in a chair facing me as we talked, and halfway through
the session I lay down and she sat on the bed beside me with her

drum, Tibetan bells, and chimes from Bali. I repeated her words as she guided me to the center of my heart, where my love for Sydney broke free. I let the words move inward as Aleta began pounding her drum loud and fast. The sound went straight to my solar plexus, resonating me to the core. Through my tears I saw Sydney running with joy, sleek and healthy as she was in her prime, with sunshine sparkling in her eyes. I knew she was free and happy and I smiled through my tears. With my heart wide open, my sadness melted into gratitude for having had so many years with her, my trusted buddy who was always up for a hike or a run and seemed to know what I was thinking or feeling before I did.

Being in that space with Aleta is like being with the Great Mother. No matter what I bring to a session, nothing can compete with the unconditional love that radiates in that room.

Opening up to receive healing is using what Aleta calls our magnetic feminine energy. This "receiving," "being" energy is different than our "doing," "giving," "go-go-go" energy she calls alpha or dynamic energy.[4] Magnetic energy draws to us what we desire and intend for our lives. We need both for a balanced, healthy life, but our culture makes it easy to get caught up in dynamic, "make it happen" energy and become alpha females who ignore the power of their receptive, allowing side. For me, Aleta's teachings about these two forces align with the essence of yoga as a pathway for balancing our energies. It's not easy—it's a daily struggle to stay with our intentions and practices, and sometimes we need a refresher course. That's why I go back to Aleta for refreshers on balancing my energies.

---

4   Aleta St. James, *Life Shift: Let Go and Live Your Dream*. Simon & Schuster, 2005, p. 52.

BENEFITS OF PERSONAL RITUALS

Scientists have discovered that humans engaged in rituals long before they began religious practices. Rituals run deep in our social DNA for a purpose—they give us a sense of control when situations seem uncontrollable. We can't control the death of a loved one, but a funeral service brings structure and order that makes us regain a sense of control. This feeling reduces our stress and anxiety, which is a win for our physical and psychological wellbeing.

Rituals affects us at the core with their meanings expressed through symbols. We create them to protect ourselves from letting fear, anxiety, and other negative emotions overwhelm us. They buffer us from the negative feedback loop that evolved to keep us on alert for danger. That drive for survival makes sense, but as behavioral scientist Nick Hobson explains:

> Since evolution is so obsessed with survival, it plays tricks on our brain. It convinces us that things are far worse than they actually are. It creates feedback cycles that force us into negative thinking patterns. The unconscious [tells us] to be extra vigilant in the event that we come across something bad…. Back in the cavewoman days it was sabre-toothed [sic] tigers. And though we no longer have to worry about these prehistoric beasts, our brain thinks we still do.[5]

The world is still a chaotic place, but rituals restore a feeling of personal order. By shutting down the negative-emotions loop, a ritual can "carry tremendous psychological and biological ben-

---

5   Nick Hobson, "The Emerging Science of Ritual: A New Look on an Ancient Behavior." *Thrive Global,* December 7, 2017. https://thriveglobal.com/stories/the-emerging-science-of-ritual-a-new-look-on-an-ancient-behavior/

efits."[6] This ties in with Kabbalah's wisdom that we should avoid the negative thought spiral and instead focus on positive emotions and being proactive. Scientists have also found that performing rituals with others makes us feel unified and trusting—the sense that we're feeling the same emotions as those around us is powerful energy. I have experienced this on every trip as we pass around the ritual talking stick and enter a place of trust and compassion for each other.

The scientific evidence invites us to bring ritual into our everyday lives to fend off our inner chatter and feel more secure. Why not create an altar, set some items on it, and repeat a few words and actions at some point every day? This simple ritual could bring a relaxing, satisfying feeling of order and control. Selecting objects that represent the four elements, for example, could be grounding and meaningful because they are tied to the natural world that we depend upon. In this corner of your world, you have the say of what is happening, when it happens, and how.

I believe that personal rituals also remind us that our intentions are in the right place. When we take the time to do a simple ritual or meditate, we are honoring our lives. We are setting an intention to bring peace, harmony, and order into our mind and body so we can be our best self when we're out in the world. Without setting intentions, we just react and swerve from one situation to another. But as I've learned from some of my favorite teachers, just stopping to think about our intentions can be transformational.

SETTING INTENTIONS WITH GRACE

Tara Brach teaches that "where intention flows, energy goes." In any situation that involves some tension, such as talking to someone who makes you feel defensive, we have an opportunity

---

6   Ibid.

to stand back and look at our intention in the moment. This is an important step—paying attention to our intention instead of just reacting. Is our intention to correct the person, tell them they are wrong? That intention may be fear based. If our broader intention is to become aligned with love in everything we do, we can choose another. "How do we open up our intention and deepen it when we are caught in a kind of egoic place?" Brach asks us. "How do we move from an ego-intention to a more spiritual intention?"[7] On this path, we pay attention and keep diving down to find our deepest intention. We ask ourselves, what is my intention right now? Is my intention to be openhearted? It sounds simple, but stopping to reflect on this is a profound practice.

Deepak Chopra also describes intentions as paths to understanding ourselves more deeply. "For every intention, we might well ask, 'How would this serve me and how would it serve everybody I come into contact with?' If the answer is that it will bring fulfillment and joy to yourself and everyone your actions impact, the intention will manifest."[8] When our desires move beyond making ourselves happy by getting things, we have a chance to find real happiness. He also writes that the "intention of the universal spirit" shows up in the form of coincidences. We sense that there is a special meaning when two things happen at the same time as if they were arranged, but appear to happen by chance. The deeper part of us knows the meaning of the coincidence, Chopra says. "Coincidences are messages from the nonlocal realm, guiding us in the ways to act in order to make our dreams, our intentions manifest."[9] He sees coincidences as the universe's way of nudging us toward our destiny.

---

7   "Tara Brach on Realizing Your Deepest Intention," YouTube, January 19, 2019.
      https://www.youtube.com/watch?v=vQHvUVZNIR4&ab_channel=TaraBrach
8   Deepak Chopra, The Spontaneous Fulfillment of Desire. Rodale, 2003, p. 112.
9   Ibid, p. 121.

Author Lynne McTaggart, who set out to research why spiritual healing works, eventually ran large experiments to explore the power of group intentions to heal. She shares solid evidence that small and large groups can heal illnesses and conditions of all kinds. Group intention work not only heals the "target" people, but also brings seemingly miraculous healing to group members themselves. Early in her experiments, she writes:

> No matter where we were in the world, in every workshop we ran, no matter how large or small, whenever we set up our clusters of eight or so people in each group, gave them a little instruction and asked them to send intention to a group member, we were stunned witnesses to the same experience: story after story of extraordinary improvement and physical and psychic transformation.[10]

McTaggart teaches how to set up "Power of Eight" groups to bring together eight people to target others for healing, and she also writes about using intentions to heal your own life. The irony of it is, your intentions are most powerful "the moment you stop thinking about yourself." Just like Tara Brach and Deepak Chopra, she has seen how intentions to serve others bring the ultimate good to everyone.

I believe that when we are intentional in everything from our choice of words to the purpose of our life goals, we take a proactive approach that keeps us open to whatever the universe has in store. Instead of resisting through negativity, we can allow our best intentions to move us through our challenges and come out better on the other side. As my Kabbalah teacher Eliyahu Jian says, we need to accept responsibility for our own evolution as human and spiritual beings. It's intentional inner work.

---

10   Lynne McTaggart, *The Power of Eight.* Simon & Schuster, 2018, p. 8.

"Religion is based on the outside that will come and save you," he said. "Spirituality is based on *you* need to save you. It's taking a lot of responsibility when you think it's you. Can you imagine if it's you, how much change you're going to make?"[11]

◌

FOR REFLECTION

1. What are your power words that define your values and priorities?

2. When did you most recently use your magnetic feminine energy?

3. Envision a space where you could set up a daily ritual. List the objects you would choose for your altar and what they symbolize. What actions and/or words would you use?

4. What is your intention for the rest of your day? For your life? As Mary Oliver asks, "What is it you plan to do with your one wild and precious life?"[12]

---

11   Stephan Spencer, "Unlock the Secrets of Your Soul with Eliyahu Jian," *Get Yourself Optimized* [podcast], February 22, 2018. https://www.getyourselfoptimized.com/unlock-secrets-soul-eliyahu-jian/
12   Mary Oliver, p. 316.

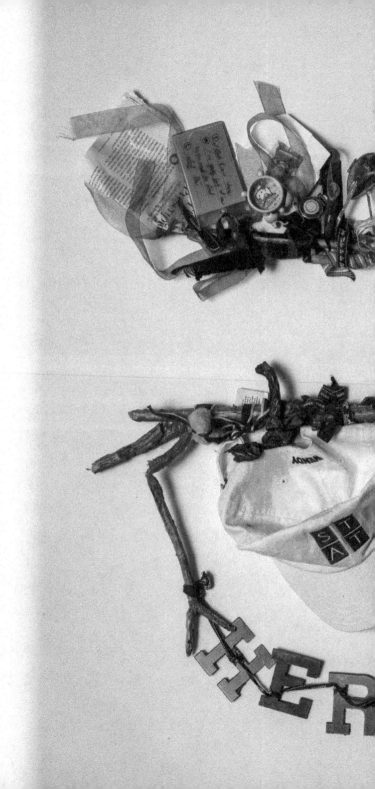

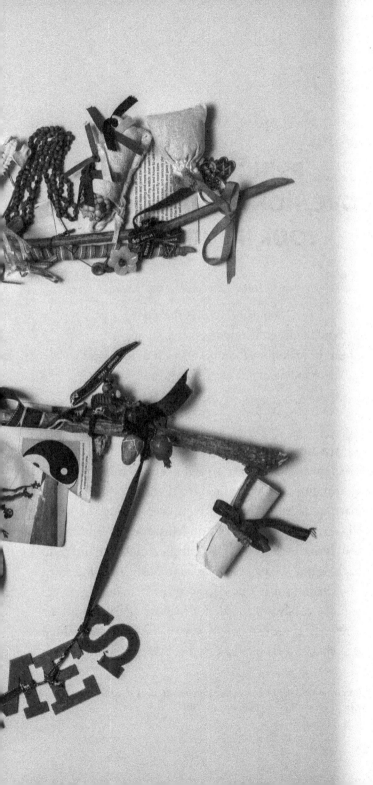

CHAPTER 9

PRINCIPLE VI: LOVE, HONOR, AND OBEY YOUR INTUITION

It is intuition that improves the world,
not just following the trodden path of thought....
The heart of man through intuition leads us to greater
understanding of ourselves and the universe.

—ALBERT EINSTEIN[1]

THERE I WAS, MINDING MY own business on a chairlift with Paul, headed up Aspen Highlands on a bright winter morning. Out of the blue, my gut told me something I didn't want to hear. We were chatting about which run we'd take among the many choices awaiting us up ahead. "Let's do Mushroom," Paul said. I hesitated, watching the sunlight blast off his sunglasses and onto mine and back again. We had done this famously long and steep trail before—Mushroom is one of the most demanding slopes anywhere—and I've always loved it. Imagine standing on the roof of the World Trade Center in a pair of skis and looking down. That's what it feels like to take off down this run, which

---

1   Albert Einstein and William Hermanns, *Einstein and the Poet: In Search of the Cosmic Man*. Branden Books, 1983, pp. 16, 109.

is nearly the same length as the span from the WTC rooftop to the street. It's a run for confident skiers that shoots between pine trees and swipes your stomach into your throat as you fly over sections that max out at thirty-six degrees steep.

I'm usually game for a thrill ride like Mushroom, but that day, something inside me shouted, *No!* I didn't want to disappoint Paul, but it just didn't feel right. I thought about it for another minute and finally said, "You know, I don't think I'm up for Mushroom today." He was okay with that, and we took the wider and less steep Scarlett's run instead. Fast forward later in the day, we read on the front page of the *Aspen News* that two skiers got caught in an avalanche on Mushroom. A crew was searching for them. The next day we learned that the pair had been found and were OK, but I still get a chill up my spine when I think about the urgent message my body gave me that day. Who knows what may have happened if I hadn't paid attention to it?

The dictionary defines intuition as *a natural ability or power that makes it possible to know something without any proof or evidence: a feeling that guides a person to act a certain way without fully understanding why.*[2] I agree that gut feelings are natural, mysterious, and persuasive. Sometimes there's a fine line between an intuitive message and a solid-sounding idea that feels so "right" we confidently go ahead with it. Choices need to be made in life, so we constantly trust that the choices we make are the right ones. Sometimes they are, but if they're not, we have to live with the consequences. Making mistakes is as natural to the human experience as having intuition. As screenwriter Charlie Kaufman says, "Failure is a badge of honor: it means you risked failure. If you don't risk failure you're never going to do anything that's

---

2   Merriam-Webster Dictionary, https://www.merriam-webster.com/dictionary/intuition

different than what you've already done, or what somebody else has done." [3]

Intuition plays into my principle that we start moving forward by making an effort, and then when we've done our best, opening up to let grace take over. I make a well-thought-out plan for a trip, then rely on grace to make it work. Along the way, my antennae are up, always ready for "gut" signals for how to proceed when the unexpected comes up.

I often feel that my intuition is fired up from the beginning, nudging me toward a particular destination. Myanmar, formerly Burma, was slowly appearing on the tourism radar when I took a group of thirteen women there in 2013, and I felt strongly drawn to it. A small window of opportunity for visitors opened in 2011 when a democratic government replaced the country's long military rule and then closed up the year after our trip due to violence between ethnic groups. The timing of our journey was remarkable, and I truly believe my intuition led me to this beautiful country.

In addition to hosting a traditional Buddhist novitiation festival for ten children and their village, we visited some of the country's most spectacular natural wonders like Inle Lake, a freshwater paradise high in the hills. Circled by mountains, the lake holds tall floating plants and fish found nowhere else in the world, and locals row their boats standing up with one leg tucked around the oar. That region's untouched beauty is beyond anything I've ever seen, but it was just one piece of Myanmar's magic. At the start of our trip we visited the twenty-six-hundred-year-old Shwedagon Pagoda, one of the oldest Buddhist temples in the world, rising from the Yangon city skyline like a gold bell with a diamond-en-

---

3   "Inspirational Writing Advice from Charlie Kaufman," Aerogramme Writers' Studio, June 12, 2019. https://www.aerogrammestudio.com/2019/06/12/inspirational-writing-advice-from-charlie-kaufman-video/

crusted spire. The Shwedagon is most famously known as a shrine, as it holds physical relics of Siddhartha Gautama Buddha, the founder of Buddhism, and three more recent Buddhas. The force of that history and eons of pilgrimages and worship hit us like a cyclone. This historic temple accepted five thousand pilgrims a day, and we were thirteen of them.

I trace the role of intuition in my travels back to my decision as a Miami girl to apply to Boston University without any outside guidance. My parents didn't even know I applied until I got in. My intuition said, *Remember how much you loved summer school in Andover outside Boston? Go back, spend four years in a real college town.* Boston may be a city of 685,000, but like New York, it's a collection of neighborhoods that makes it feel like a town. My decision to go abroad to London for junior year was another jump into the unknown that gave me the travel bug that would ultimately turn into STAT. Throughout my life, trusting my intuition has helped me become my own best advocate.

WHITE-COLLAR INTUITION

Intuition is also alive and well in the corporate business world. The majority of top-level executives rely on their intuition as well as facts when making decisions.[4] They may not talk about it, but these leaders credit their intuition for "eureka" moments that spring up during a stressful decision-making process—in an instant, the mind taps into an underground pool of wisdom based on years of experience and learning. Having a competitive edge with "intuitiveness," they say, relies on a foundation of experience and knowledge, being open and curious, and having

---

4   Jay Liebowitz, "Intuition-based Decision-making: The Other Side of Analytics." Analytics, March 2, 2015. https://pubsonline.informs.org/do/10.1287/LYTX.2015.02.02/full/

the courage to act on gut-feeling hunches.[5] Sir Richard Branson famously followed his intuition to go into the airline industry in 1984, ignoring the "logical" advice of his friends and colleagues who insisted it was a bad idea. As we all know, Virgin Airlines was a huge success.

Steve Jobs, cofounder of Apple, is another business legend renowned for his intuitive thinking. In an interview, Jobs explained how studying Buddhism took him down this path: "I began to realize that an intuitive understanding and consciousness was more significant than abstract thinking and intellectual logical analysis.... I'm one of the few people who understands how producing technology requires intuition and creativity."[6] Six years before his death, Jobs famously advised Stanford University grads to value their intuition in his 2005 commencement address:

> Don't be trapped by dogma—which is living with the results of other people's thinking. Don't let the noise of others' opinions drown out your own inner voice. And most important, have the courage to follow your heart and intuition. They somehow already know what you truly want to become. Everything else is secondary.[7]

I like the idea that people we assume are totally right-brained and logical, like CEOs of big corporations, have figured out that intuition is valuable, even priceless. Who knew that a globe-trotting entrepreneur like Branson or tech wizard like Jobs have some-

5   G. J. Koshy, K. A. April, & B. Dharani, B. (2020). Intuition and Decision-Making: Business and Sports Leaders. *Effective Executive, 23*(2), 31-65. https://www-proquest-com.ezproxy.mnsu.edu/scholarly-journals/intuition-decision-making-business-sports-leaders/docview/2446289840/se-2?accountid=12259

6   Walter Isaacson, Steve Jobs. Simon & Schuster, 2013, pp. 35, 397.

7   "'You've got to find what you love,' Jobs says," *Stanford News*, June 14, 2005. https://news.stanford.edu/2005/06/14/jobs-061505/

thing precious in common with my childhood friend, Nancy, who also changes the world with her intuition, one person at a time?

INTUITION OFF THE CHARTS

Nancy Torgove Clasby has always had a strong intuition. For her, intuition is the understanding that we are all connected, and throughout her life she has experienced those connections in fascinating ways that have always felt natural and "organically normal." In her book, *The Reluctant Mystic: Autobiography of an Awakening*, she tells the story of being reconnected with her grandmother shortly after she died. Nancy was three years old when she heard the phone ring, answered it in her tiny hands, and heard her grandmother tell her she was okay and that she loved her. The call seemed so natural, their connection so unaffected by death, that Nancy never told anyone about it. Years later, after she was married and the mother of three young children, Nancy had a transcendent awakening experience that changed her life forever. Blissfully immersed in an all-knowing, all-loving, all-powerful light, she had "an inner knowing and sureness that everything is exactly the way it is supposed to be" and that "we are all connected."[8] After her awakening, she could see energy fields in people and other living things, understand the meaning of human existence, and heal people of cancer and other ailments. She shared with me that her perspective of life embraces the Jewish teaching that "the veil is closed over our eyes when we're born, and life is about pulling that veil up and learning who we are, what our challenges are, and what we're here to do."

---

8   Nancy Torgove Clasby, *The Reluctant Mystic: Autobiography of an Awakening*, Small Batch Books, 2016, p. 8–9.

For Nancy, we all tap into our intuition at different levels, and this aspect of our soul can answer the big questions about our unique gifts and purpose:

For some the gift can be small: a grateful heart, generosity, a smile. When you're around a generous person, it's a wonderful gift. Not everyone can do what Erin does, but she can because she's strong, open hearted, and has a body that won't give up on any level and a spirit that swirls around her, saying, let's do this! Her spirit tickles the imagination. She learned this was her gift.

Nancy also believes the key to intuition is using the body to slow down and listen:

Intuition is tied into our lives in different ways—there are as many ways to intuit as there are human beings on the planet. We find our intuition in the present moment. That's why the great mystical traditions use breathing, which brings us into the present moment. All the mysteries of the world are in our breath. When we focus on our breath through meditation, yoga, or qigong, we slow down the body, open the heart center, and connect to our higher power.

Nancy's story of awakening inspires me to stay curious about the mysteries of life and to trust that all is well, always. Her gifts of healing and awareness show us what intuition looks like at the highest level, off the charts and capable of miracles.

On a STAT trip to Peru, my friend Jodi, the therapeutic yoga expert who led our yoga sessions on several trips, felt her intuition working overtime. The day we explored Machu Picchu, she branched off on her own and sensed a distinct energy in each space. Machu Picchu, built in a hidden niche in the Andes in the fifteenth century, is believed to have been a retreat for Inca royalty. None of us were surprised when the magnificent compound of residences, temples, and stepped terraces was aptly named one of the "New Seven Wonders of the World" in 2007. As Jodi walked among the ruins, she felt different energies in each structure. In the Palace of the Incas, for example, she had a strong impression that women had stayed and felt trapped in the many small rooms in the building, but her sensation of the Temple of the Sun was blissfully positive. "At every turn I felt a different energy," she said.

To her amazement, Jodi's intuitive encounter with Machu Picchu's energies was topped the next day by her experience in our session with a local shaman. "When you work with a shaman," she said, "they can really push you over your borderline, and I love it." The shaman had us lying on the stone ground as he drummed and chanted with his ceremonial objects. His English was spotty, but we didn't seem to need detailed instructions anyway, his ritual pulled us into another state of consciousness. The otherworldly atmosphere of Machu Picchu itself may have also played a part. He told us to imagine our bodies sinking deep into the Earth while our souls lifted into the sky, and Jodi felt a sharp awareness of both at the same time. "I've done a lot of crazy shit," she said, "but I never felt anything like that before. I became totally weightless. I had a completely new sense of being." We each felt transported in our way. I believe letting go is easier when you are surrounded by people you trust.

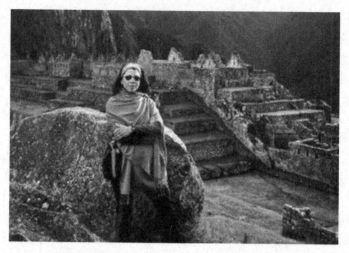

A solitary moment in Machu Picchu. *(Photo: Author's Archive)*

Stories throughout this book have described how the therapy part of my Sports Travel Adventure Therapy trips for women often weaves around the bond we make as a group. Hiking, climbing, biking, rowing, doing yoga, eating, drinking, and participating in spiritual ceremonies together builds up an energy field unique to each group. This rare environment is ripe with opportunities for change, within and without. I believe we sometimes get an intuitive inkling about an upcoming transformative experience, a hint that change is on the way. My friend and longtime STAT traveler Jen felt this before a trip to Sedona that coincided with her fortieth birthday. She recognized that she was not in a marriage that was going to last forever, and beneath the surface, every emotional button around divorce was getting pushed. She knew that a STAT trip, with its heart-opening rituals and opportunities to talk, would bring her underlying tensions, worries, and realizations to the fore. "My intuition was that I was going to walk out of there a different person," she said. "I had a sense of change but didn't know what it would look like."

Jen's conflicted thoughts about leaving a marriage and upending the rules and expectations that had always defined her percolated throughout the trip. By the last night, she was ready for a gift of clarity:

> We advanced to our final night with the sweat lodge ceremony. It was there, thanks to Native American psychotherapy, if you will, that I saw what I needed to do. Like on a vision quest, I had clarity to own what I was and where I was going, to accept that I couldn't see the outcome but knew what I was heading toward. The sense of intuition also played out in terms of Erin's ability to hit the nail on the head in terms of what we needed— especially what I needed: to find my voice. This is often a struggle for women. My parents had high expectations for me, but I was still the girl. I have a big voice, literally, and that was encouraged, but I also felt I was trapped in this model of "You stay with one person your whole life." That night, I was finally able to start to let that go.

Jen's path to freeing herself from expectations and models that no longer worked for her was a long one, taking a few years. Maybe attachments we've supported our entire lives are sewn in so firmly they take a while to loosen. There is a lot to learn along the way, of course, which is the whole point. About five years later, on our STAT trip to Cambodia and Laos, being far from home and all things familiar gave Jen the space to feel how far she'd come in untying those threads. "That trip was an intimate, extraordinary experience," she said. "I knew when I arrived that I was heading to the final chapter of my marriage." On one level, she told me, she felt an incredible sense of freedom from being bound by society's and her own pressures of what marriage is supposed to be, and that freedom opened the door to "a tremendous amount of intuition about ending my marriage," she said.

As we hiked through a Cambodian rainforest, Jen relied on the security of the group and her sense of adventure to carry her through her fear of snakes. This part of the world is, after all, home to big boys like king cobras, pythons, and 150-pound anacondas. As she made her way along the trail, she was surprised that her fear didn't grip her. Her expanding sense of freedom was feeding into her overall boldness about life, giving her more control over her fear. This awareness fit with other changes she'd made by then, including launching her radio show, "A Fashionable Life," and moving much closer to ending her marriage. She had hit her stride in finding her voice and gained a broader perspective, which in Cambodia helped her size up her problems in a new way. "In Cambodia, you're exposed to the history of the killing fields," she said. "There's suffering, and there's *that* suffering. It gave me the clarity I needed at that time."

For Jen, finding her voice also meant giving her sense of humor free reign. Every STAT trip reminds me that humor is important when the going gets a little rough, and Cambodia was no exception. One day, after kayaking down the Mekong Delta and hiking in the blasted humidity, we arrived at a cave carved into a mountain. Standing in a circle, our socks soaked through inside our rubber Teva shoes, we listened to the woman guide tell us about the Buddhist figures scattered among the lit candles around the cave. Jen felt something on her ankle—"As a former *Vogue* editor," she reminded me later, "those Tevas were so against my style"—and looked down at her feet. There was blood:

A big black leech was crawling out the top of my foot. That explained the blood all over my socks and the freaked-out look on everybody's face. I'm a diffuser, so

I pointed around the circle and said, "*None* of you can *ever* refer to me as a JAP (Jewish American Princess)! We all exploded into laughter. When we walked out to get our ride, I ceremoniously pulled off my shoes and leechy socks and tossed them in the little garbage can outside the cave.

By the time she was fifty, Jen had gotten divorced and was happily remarried with two lovely stepchildren. Years later, she joined our group who traveled to the middle-of-nowhere West Texas town of Marfa—the desert spot that Donald Judd, the foremost American minimalist sculptor, put on the map—for Marjorie's sixtieth birthday celebration. "It's hard to get here, but everyone's welcome," seems to be the Marfa mantra. We stayed at the historic Cibolo Creek Ranch, just outside Marfa with its single traffic light that always blinks yellow. Surrounded by the Chinati and Cienega Mountains, Marfa was the perfect backdrop for taking stock. At night we gathered by the campfire under an unbelievably starry Texas sky to break out in song and talk about life, death, transcendence, and self-reflection. Nothing but wading into the deep end in that group.

It's hard to describe surrealistic, bizarre Marfa, where Jen said she felt "so in my body." That trip served as kind of a check of where she had started and how far she'd come. Our women's adventure trips, she said, "provided the significant points on our evolution from our forties to fifties, a great road map for our maturation, acceptance, and always ceding to intuition first, not allowing outside pressures and shame to get in the way of our truth and our voice."

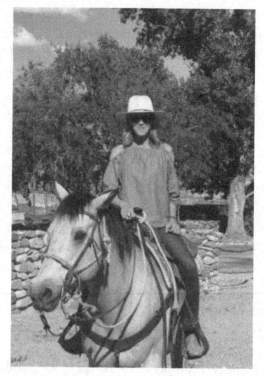

Jen in the saddle in Marfa. *(Photo: Author's Archive)*

In Marfa, we kept finding ourselves smack in the middle of metaphors, like gorgeous fusions of the ultramodern with the old and horse rides into the sunset. Nothing could be further from our bustling, ordinary lives, and that was the plan. The thing is, every town or home has its own Marfa, a space we can find or carve out for ourselves that invites us to sit down, breathe, and go within. We all need a quiet space, a room of our own, and our intuition can help us find it and bring us deeper when we get there.

ℛ

FOR REFLECTION

1. How do you feel your "gut" messages? In your stomach, heart, as an electric charge, hearing a voice, something else?

2. What is your most memorable experience with your intuition?

3. What stories have you heard about a friend or relative being protected or otherwise guided by their intuition?

4. If you're a parent, have you talked to your child about intuition? How did the subject come up?

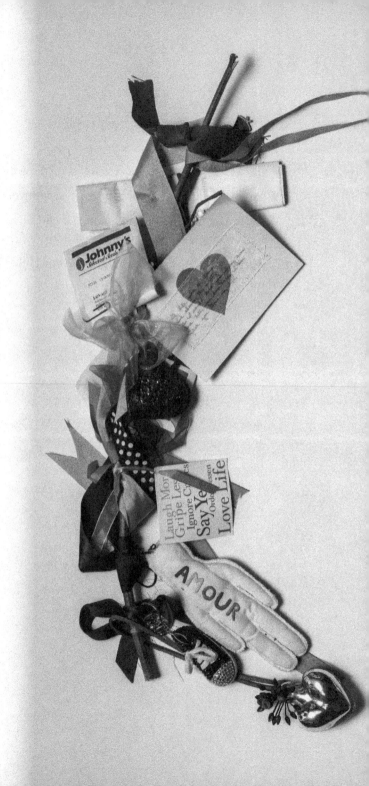

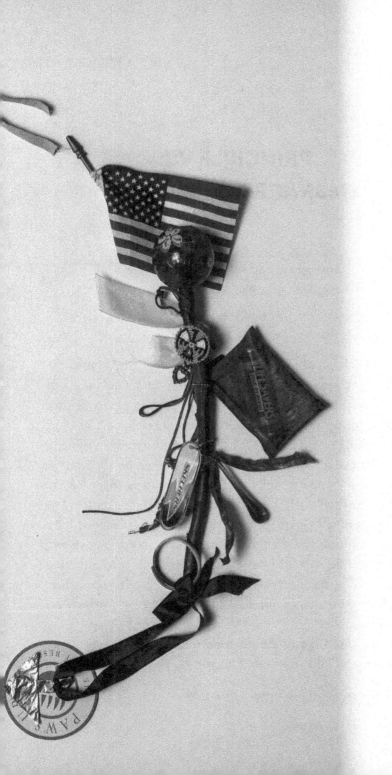

CHAPTER 10

PRINCIPLE VII: EMBRACE COMMUNITY

*Connection, along with love and belonging
(two expressions of connection), is why we are here.*

—Brené Brown[1]

EARLY ON SEPTEMBER 11, 2001, I was driving into Manhattan for a doctor's appointment. My boys were in school near our home in Connecticut, and I knew I'd get back in plenty of time to pick them up in the afternoon. The sky was a perfect blue, but everything else felt weird. A plume of smoke was visible in the far distance in lower Manhattan. As I parked on the street, a news bulletin came on the radio saying that a passenger jet had crashed into the North Tower of the World Trade Center. The reporters were talking about a possible accident. I listened for a couple of minutes and then started walking to my appointment, joining the street vibe of mass confusion. People were gathering outside storefronts and apartment buildings to talk, and others were glued to their cell phones. Everyone looked worried, off kilter, vulnerable.

By the time I got to the doctor's office, panic had set in the waiting room. "Did you hear? Did you *hear*?" a nurse asked me.

---

1   Brené Brown, *Daring Greatly*. Avery, 2012, p. 68.

"Two planes hit the World Trade Center! Both towers!" The half dozen or so of us standing around stared at each other. What could it be? What's happening? Sirens started going off all over the place outside and I clicked into mother mode. No one knew what was going on, but two hits to the World Trade Center were no accident. I had to get back to Connecticut and pick up my boys. Paul was in Atlanta on business, so I was on my own.

When I finally got to my car and started driving toward the Triborough Bridge, I came up against a row of orange cones at an intersection blocking my way. People were rushing around, sirens were blasting. It looked like a barricade was being set up around the city, but I had to get out. Jacked up on adrenalin, I jumped out of the car and kicked away the cones so I could keep driving toward the bridge. All the way home the radio reports grew more disturbing and I was sure I wasn't the only one wondering if New York would get hit again. Every cell in my body felt connected to every person, place, and thing in the city. The oneness I felt in my heart for the city came through the icy shock and felt primal, territorial. Every New Yorker I know, especially those who were in town that day, describes this feeling in their own way. Our bond with the city, something so much larger than ourselves, connected us like family.

Nineteen years later, this sense of oneness was front and center again in the first weeks of COVID. Pent-up New Yorkers improvised their way into a beautiful display of pride in our city. At 7:00 p.m. every evening, people opened their windows and clanged on pans to salute the doctors, nurses, and other healthcare workers who were risking their lives on the front lines. I missed this ritual after we left for Colorado to wait out the pandemic—I felt I'd abandoned my city in the worst of times. I would call my friends at 7:00 p.m. and ask them to hold their phones outside the window so I could hear the pounding of the pans. At a time when we all needed the comfort of connection—the bigger the community, the better—I felt wrenched away from my eight-million-person-strong tribe.

When vaccines became available in 2021, we were back in New York and I signed up to get a shot at the Javits Convention Center on the West Side. Hundreds of us moved through the lines in that gigantic space packed with Army volunteers and healthcare practitioners administering shots. I was so proud of the efficient organization of it all and felt that special bond that comes with doing your civic duty.

People are hardwired for connection. We're deeply social beings. This is why my community of STAT clients is my lifeline—for nearly three decades I have felt the power of bonding that takes place over the course of a few days and sends us back to our everyday lives with more confidence and deeper connections. Sociologist and author Brené Brown says connection is the energy we create between each other when we feel "seen, heard, and valued" and can be ourselves without feeling judged. That's exactly how we feel on our adventure travels, so open and vulnerable from pushing ourselves physically that our conversations and rituals let our truth flow, free of judgments. Belonging, Brené says, is something different—the primal desire to be part of something greater than ourselves. Needing to belong is not an ego thing, but part of the fiber of being human, and it's spiritual. As Brené said in an interview on Krista Tippet's "On Being":

> At the very heart of belonging is spirituality—not religion, not dogma, but spirituality...the deeply held belief that we're inextricably connected to each other by something greater than us. And that thing that is greater than us is rooted in love and compassion—that there's some-

thing bigger than us and that we are connected to each other in a way that cannot be severed.[2]

This helps explain my feelings after 9/11; my sense of belonging—that spiritual sense of being part of something larger than myself—was crushed because the "something" I belonged to was fractured. At the same time, I felt my connection to the city more deeply than ever before. The pain and the love were mixed together. As a rule, I feel part of something bigger than myself in everything I do. The universe has so many messages about something bigger than me. I know without a doubt that I'm part of something bigger, and I love that feeling. I keep my friends close and connected, but I also like to be alone. I've found the right balance, and I hope I have instilled in my sons these priorities for healthy relationships, community, giving and receiving love, and having a sense of purpose.

Our spiritual instinct to connect and belong leads us to people who help us feel whole and alive. How many times have you met someone and both of you feel that you have known each other forever? Our close friendships may be few in number, but they are our lifeblood, literally! Friendship is a gift that goes a long way, because the positive feedback loop of feeling connected with others touches every area of our health.

Decades of medical research tell us that friendship and social connection boosts the immune system, speeds up recovery time when we get sick, and adds years to our lives. Having friends improves cancer survival, lowers the risk of heart disease, relieves some of the symptoms of depression and posttraumatic stress disorder, controls blood sugar levels, and protects us from the harm of unhealthy habits like smoking and avoiding exercise. Our

---

2   Krista Tippett, "Brené Brown, : Strong Back, Soft Front, Wild Heart." On Being with Krista Tippet, January 2, 2020.

bodies reward us for personal connections by releasing the feel-good hormone oxytocin when we hug, hold hands, get a massage, and have sexual intimacy.[3] Without social connection, the opposite is true. An alienated life not only brings on loneliness that can lead to depression, but also damages our physiology. We know that *social isolation is more harmful to our health than smoking, high blood pressure, and obesity.*[4] We need each other, from head to toe.

CONNECTING GREATLY

Each of my women's adventure trips has formed its own community of openness and trust. We keep proving Brené Brown's message that "the foundation of courage is vulnerability—the ability to navigate uncertainty, risk, and emotional exposure."[5] In the safe circle of the group, our energy doesn't go to seeking approval or trying to fit in. Our natural inclination is to be our vulnerable, imperfect selves. As my friend Susan M. recalled, even when most women in a group have never met before, the rituals and outdoor workouts bring out our vulnerability and, as a result, draw everyone together:

> When you become vulnerable and talk about the most difficult thing you're going through in life, change happens. On day three, after you've done the talking stick ceremony the night before, everyone starts to talk about how they can relate to someone's story. We share more

---

3   Martino et al., "The Connection Prescription," *Analytic Review,* 2015. https://www.ncbi.nlm.nih.gov/pmc/articles/PMC6125010/

4   Emma Seppälä, "Social Connection Boosts Health, Even When You're Isolated," *Psychology Today,* March 23, 2020.

5   Brené Brown, "Why Experiencing Joy and Pain in a Group Is So Powerful." *Greater Good Magazine,* January 9, 2019. https://greatergood.berkeley.edu/article/item/why_experiencing_joy_and_pain_in_a_group_is_so_powerful

about what we know and how we may be able to help. If you take advantage of being true and honest, this starts to open up a whole slew of changes. At this stage in my life I crave female companionship. It's so comforting to be with other women. I think that as we get older, women are drawn to book clubs or tennis or other activities to be with other women. Our children are grown and we're all going through many of the same things at the same time. We're drawn to that community, and that female bonding is a large part of what Erin does for women by creating these trips.

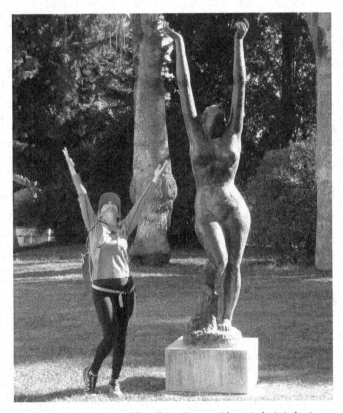

Susan M. feeling the goddess vibe in Croatia. *(Photo: Author's Archive)*

Donna, who has also been on several STAT trips, remembers the positive impact of our little community on a journey that took place during a rough time in her life. "On the Morocco trip," she said, "I had just lost my younger brother, who I was very close to. I felt compelled to share about that, and processing how I felt was very hard, but I got so much compassion from those women that it was a very healing experience for me." Several of the women on these trips can be total strangers, she said, but an open and nonjudgmental attitude, being "real and vulnerable," puts everyone on equal footing. "People open up," she said.

Donna told me that her most physically challenging STAT trip was to Tasmania and Australia, where we hiked more than forty miles a day with twenty-pound backpacks. She trusted me, the two women guides I hired, and the power of the group energy to get her through. "I have a very small frame, so that physical part was extremely challenging for me," she said. "It took more than physical fitness to deal with the rock climbing, changing temperatures, and sheer length of the days; it was about having grit and determination." She couldn't imagine what it would have been like without being okay with her vulnerability:

> I had to feel vulnerable because here we were in this very open terrain and living with the bare essentials. It made you realize what you can live without—I didn't miss a thing. Instead, it made me focus more on the beauty of everything around me. We were led by these two young girls in their early twenties, which made me realize there was a lot of trust out there. If you had a problem, the only way out was by helicopter. Those girls were so responsible and organized and had such good judgment, and we also trusted in Erin. We always put so much trust in her. That trust and everything else combined—the laughter

and physical support—happen because we're free to feel vulnerable on these trips.

Another example of successfully navigating uncertainty, one of Brené Brown's signposts of vulnerability, cropped up for my STAT client Minnie in Columbia. On the first day of our four-day hike to the ancient Lost City, fast-walking Minnie was up ahead of the group with the local guide. Soaked to the skin in the pounding rain, they began to cross a river, but the water was rising quickly. The guide sensed that the river would flood in a matter of minutes, so he quickly lifted Minnie up onto his shoulders and carried her across. On the other side, the steep clay road had already turned into a raging waterfall. The guide scrambled back across the river to get to the rest of us before we approached the flash flood. Left alone, Minnie walked over to a nearby hut and was invited in by a friendly woman and her two young children. As an experienced traveler and all-around tough chick, she took her vulnerable situation in stride and settled in with them. Meanwhile, I was worried about her as I huddled with our group in the freezing-cold rain and mud.

Although Minnie spoke very little Spanish and her hosts spoke no English, they smiled at each other and communicated with the universal language of facial expressions and gestures that travelers often resort to. "For three-and-a-half hours I just hung out with this nice lady and her two kids," Minnie said. "I told myself I was going to be OK. The rain was going to stop and they'd come find me. I'm not an anxiety-ridden person, so I relaxed and thought, 'It is what it is.'"

That's mindfulness for you.

It didn't take long to find Minnie once the rain stopped and the river tamed down. Her story and unshakable calm inspired us for the rest of that extremely challenging trip. I can control everything on a STAT trip except the weather, so I'm grateful for the way Minnie handled herself and how we all managed to stay safe amid a flood, wild weather, and steep terrain in that remote slice of Columbia.

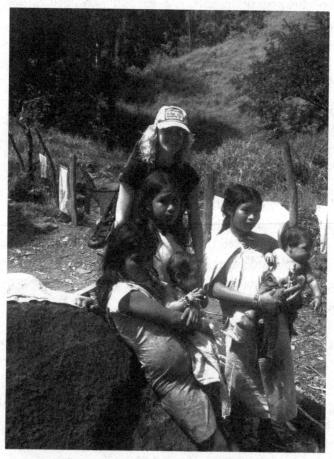

Minnie with the woman and her children (and friends) who sheltered her during a flash flood in Columbia. *(Photo: Author's Archive)*

On the lighter side, for most people, there's nothing like being naked to make you feel vulnerable. Donna and I had a good laugh about this when we were roommates on a STAT trip to Croatia, where I was surprised to learn she was so modest. As she tells the story:

> I was enjoying a bath after a long day and Erin came in and looked enviously at the tub. She always walks around naked in hotel rooms—she was born without a shame gene. She said, 'That looks nice—move over!' I told her I'd never taken a bath with a girl before, and she said, 'It's a big bathtub, move over!' She plopped in and we laughed so hard. I'm not immodest, but I'm certainly a lot less modest now than I was before going on Erin's trips.

WE CAN DO THIS

The health benefits of personal connections are amped up when our social circle also happens to be a healthy influence. Dan Buettner, author of the *Blue Zones* books about the lifestyles of the world's happiest and longest-living people, visited us in Aspen many years ago and opened our eyes to the easy ways communities can get healthier. After our week together hiking and skiing and gathering for dinner with friends, I was proud to hear Dan declare Aspen an "honorary" Blue Zone! He shared with us that the habits of everyone in our close-knit circle of friends and/or family are contagious. It's a good idea to make sure our social circles nourish us in body and mind, because "The most profound, measurable, and long-lasting thing you can do is build a social circle around yourself that supports healthy eating, activity, and emotional well-being," Dan writes.[6] Another habit common to the world's happiest people is spiritual belonging—people who

---

6   Dan Buettner, *The Blue Zones Challenge*. National Geographic, 2021. p. 48.

regularly attend religious services (faith or denomination doesn't matter), Dan's research found, outlive their life expectancy by fourteen years.

For me, it's all about balance and moderation, like the 80/20 approach to eating healthy most of the time and indulging once in a while. I'm grateful to have a close circle of friends who reinforce that view. For everyone, everywhere, gathering together and gifting ourselves with loving relationships is good medicine.

I love *New York Times* columnist and TV news commentator David Brook's story about putting meaningful connection at the center of his life. After his divorce in 2013, David was living alone in an apartment and doing nothing but work. His only friends were his job colleagues, and he described his isolated lifestyle as "being in the valley." After meeting a family whose home was full of love and dozens of kids who needed a place to stay, he was hit smack in the heart with the realization that relationship is everything. He saw the country's problems as problems of disconnection. The solution, he decided, was spreading stories and inspiration about people who put loving relationships first and offering real-world ways for anyone to do the same. He called connection-centered people "weavers" because they weave a rich social fabric in their communities, and used the name for a project he launched at the Aspen Institute. The tagline for Weave: The Social Fabric Project is "Lead with Love." David believes that small acts of love and generosity can transform our culture from one "that values achievement and individual success to one that finds value in deep relationships and community success."[7]

I see missions like Weave's as a reflection of the work many are doing within themselves, shifting from a focus on the indi-

7   Weave: The Social Fabric Project, "Why I Started Weave, An Interview with David Brooks." The Aspen Institute, 2020, https://weareweavers.org/weavers/why-i-started-weave-an-interview-with-david-brooks/

vidual to one on connection. With connection comes more room for love, the source of it all, to flow.

My greatest wish is that the women who journey out of their comfort zones and into the wild with me return home to enjoy their life and love connections a little more. May the ripples flow.

ॐ

FOR REFLECTION

1. When an experience like an illness or getting bad news makes you feel vulnerable, is there someone in your life you can count on to embrace and not judge your vulnerable, imperfect self?

2. The last time you attended a large event like a football game, concert, or wedding, what emotion did you have that you felt was shared by everyone else in the crowd?

3. How many people do you consider close friends, members of your "tribe?" How often do you get together with them? Does that feel often enough?

4. What small act of kindness could you do on your next trip to the grocery store?

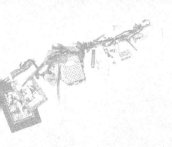
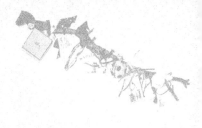

PART III

EVER MOVING ON

Nature knows best, and she says, *roar*!

—Maria Edgeworth[1]

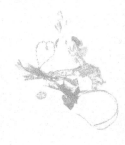

---

1   Maria Edgeworth, *Ormond: A Tale*. Macmillan, 1895, p. 46

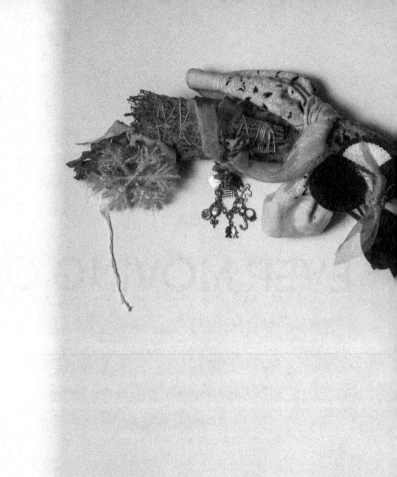

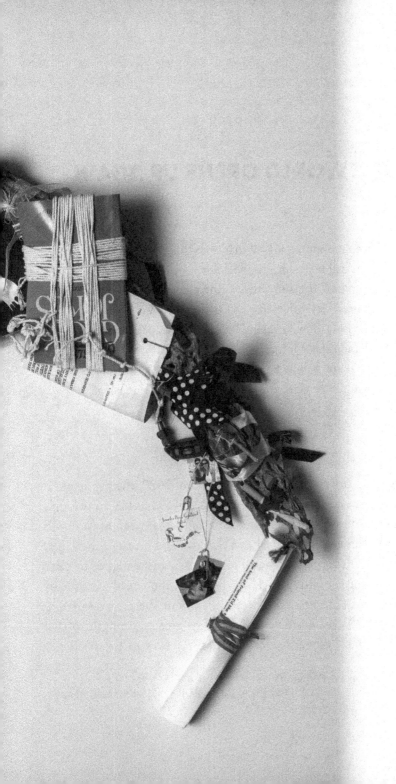

CHAPTER 11

THE WORLD OPENS UP AGAIN

I keep reminding myself that everything that 2020 has
been will make for great lockdown stories to tell later
and to look back on when we are older. I had a socially
distanced eleventh birthday. I had endless family time. I
learned how to make scrambled eggs and pancakes, banana
bread and cake from scratch. Twenty years from now, a kid
just like me will be learning about what I went through,
in a history class. And I think that's pretty amazing!

—CAROLINA CARABALLO, 11, BRONX, NEW YORK,
IN A *TIME* MAGAZINE INTERVIEW, 2021[2]

As I WRITE THIS FINAL chapter at the end of 2022, the pandemic is
waning, but not over with us yet. COVID-19 has blazed through
the world more than once, and no scientist can assure us it will
disappear forever. But I take heart that this is the Year of the Tiger,
a time for mustering our fierce and courageous energies to clear
out whatever is holding back our lives and the world—a time of
purging and renewal. For all the horrors of the past two years,
I believe COVID has given many of us greater strength to face
our challenges, especially by opening our eyes to the precious-

---

2 Jeffrey Kluger and Allison Singer, "'A Year Full of Emotions.' What Kids
Learned from the COVID-19 Pandemic," *Time,* June 12, 2021, https://time.
com/6071300/kids-pandemic/

ness of our relationships. In an era filled with illness, loss, and isolation, I learned to never take friendship or family for granted again. This insight is the flip side of suffering. As Rumi wrote, "Whenever sorrow comes, be kind to it, for God has placed a pearl in sorrow's hand."[3]

In that context, COVID was a welcome pause that brought me closer to the people I most care about. The pearl, the gift of COVID, was learning down to my bones what is really important and the beauty of being surrounded by a circle of family and friends I could always count on. To be honest—and I don't say this to be cavalier or to disregard the suffering and death of millions in our human family—as I reflect on the good that COVID brought me, I wouldn't want to have missed it.

Like thousands of others, Paul and I were hit by COVID the first year before the vaccines came out. We were sick in bed for two weeks, and I'll never forget what it felt like to be so shut down that I couldn't raise my head from my pillow. The headaches were excruciating. Being that vulnerable opened something in me, and as a result I feel privileged to live through this time. I'm now even more willing to let what comes come and not push or compete. Instead, I always remind myself, what's the rush in life? We're all going to the same place. I've seen many people come out of the COVID era with a new ability to slow down and "smell" the roses. In a time of quarantines, school closings, hospital crises, lost jobs, social isolation, illness, and death, we've spent more quality time with our friends and family by reaching out with phone and video calls and emails. We've made it a top priority to nurture our circle for the sake of emotional, physical, and soul survival.

---

3   Amit Deep Kumar, *Soul Cuppa: The Cup of Soul,* Notion Press, 2017, p. 31.

At the start of it all, when I was laid up in Aspen from a skiing accident, I got a full dose of what community really means. Locals like store and gallery owners and others I knew from being in town for over twenty years (making me almost a local) were there for me. Since I couldn't walk myself down the street let alone my dog, my dog-walking friends were so generous with their time. Even my friends in the fire department checked in on me! People dropped off things and drove me to my doctor appointments and called me to see how I was. When they called, I'd start crying and moan, "I'm not okay!" I was in never-never land, ripped from my active routines and drained of energy and the endorphins that made me feel good, energetic, and normal. It felt like my blood had stopped circulating—my active way of life was on hold, and I had no idea how to deal with it. Thank goodness my community was a poster child for lovingkindness. Two years later, people are still extra considerate. Instead of a worn-out maxim, "Love your neighbor" has become a real thing, expressed by all the small but meaningful acts we know we should do. Anyone who has been at the receiving end of such kindness knows that a little goes a long way. As the world opens up again, it seems our hearts are more willing to connect and to motivate us to walk our talk.

While putting my STAT trip plans on hold, I missed the camaraderie of my girls—my STAT tribe. Even in-country trips were out of the question throughout 2020, and rightly so. At the end of that year, U.S. domestic flights were down 59 percent compared to 2019 and the number of international flights were still inching along at 70 percent less than the year before.[4] In 2021 I cancelled my first plans for a Bolivia trip because I didn't

---

4   Bureau of Transportation Statistics, "Full-Year 2020 and December 2020
     U.S. Airline Traffic Data," March 11, 2021. https://www.bts.gov/newsroom/
     full-year-2020-and-december-2020-us-airline-traffic-data

want to put anyone at risk. Half of the women who signed up were willing to go, but the other half didn't feel comfortable. I sided with caution and, as I mentioned in Chapter 8, ultimately scheduled the trip for November 2022. Since the travel scene was looking up in the last part of 2021, I also scheduled a very special trip for May 2022.

As the pandemic loosened its grip, U.S. airlines saw an 82 percent increase in passengers in 2021 compared to 2020.[5] Many Americans were making plans to travel again and I felt fortunate to be one of them, alongside my clients. Every time I sent out a trip update email, booked a lodge, or hired a guide, a shot of endorphins sent my heart racing in anticipation. I'll have a group again! Most of us were friends, but there were also a few new faces, each of us curious about how the terrain would crash us through our comfort zones, inside and out.

When it comes to travel inside the U.S., I hope the COVID-caused surge in visits to our national parks stays on course. From Mount Rainier to the Everglades and the Badlands to Big Bend, our parks offer a lifetime of exploration. Many aspects of our lives may now be permanently different, such as working from home and using technology to regularly connect, but opportunities to trek into nature are with us as they've always been. Our cities have parks. Our suburbs have walking trails. Our small towns have rivers or lakes to fish and swim. Every part of the country carries a historic natural destination waiting for our eyes, ears, hands, and feet to behold. North America offers endless locations for trips of a lifetime, but for my let's-get-out-of-dodge spring 2022 trip, I chose to cross a few international borders.

---

5   Bureau of Transportation Statistics, "Full-Year 2021 and December 2021 U.S. Airline Traffic Data," March 10, 2022. https://www.bts.gov/newsroom/full-year-2021-and-december-2021-us-airline-traffic-data

INTO THIN AIR

I scheduled my first post-COVID-lockdown STAT trip in an extraordinary location to celebrate the world opening up again. My STAT travelers, like me, craved an adventure to challenge themselves and blast them out of their long-isolation comfort zones. In some ways, two years of isolation had starved our spirits. We needed to jump start our lives with a peak experience, like a once-in-a-lifetime mountain adventure. Where are the world's most famous heights? Nepal, of course. Home to eight of the ten tallest mountains in the world, including Everest, Nepal promised magic. And it delivered. Our journey was worth its weight in gold.

I had the great fortune of booking explorer extraordinaire Johan Ernst as our guide. Nepal held a special place in Johan's heart since he summited Everest in 2007, and when earthquakes struck during another expedition in 2015, he joined other guides and climbers in rescue and rebuild missions. Four years earlier he had led the Saving Everest Project that removed nine tons of garbage from Everest and its trails.

A Swedish explorer who has won too many awards and recognitions to mention for his environmental activism and philanthropic work (most recently the 2022 Activist of the Year award at the Cannes Film Festival), Johan is not your typical guide. Before signing on with me, he wanted to know my purpose, my gut reason for taking eleven women to trek the Himalayas (Everest wasn't our goal—as tens of thousands of other mere mortals know, there are many other climbs in these mountains with Everest often in view). An adventure trip, Johan said, is about what it's going to mean to other people, not just you personally. He believes there's a higher purpose in everything you do in life, and giving back is part of his philosophy. He was happy to learn that I shared the same outlook and included philanthropy in all my trips, and I think he was especially intrigued by the idea of leading his first all-woman trip. We were honored by this opportunity to trek with one of the most famous explorers in the world who was considered family to many villagers and Sherpas in Nepal.

Johan's definition of the three phases of an adventure trip also lined up with my own. He explained that the first is when you plan, dream, train, prepare, and organize. Next is when you live in the moment with the adventure while exploring and experiencing the incredible scenery and challenging terrain, in this case hiking in high altitudes. Then we take the memories home with us, which is where we learn to share and understand the life-changing adventure to the Top of the World. We were totally in synch on this. Check, check, and check.

With the COVID threat still alive and other chaos spiraling in the world, everything was so unpredictable while planning this trip and starting out. What if someone got COVID at the last minute? What if a new surge made it impossible for us to leave Nepal? Fortunately, I sighed with relief that first night—everybody made it! Then, getting to the first lodge, everybody made it! Not even a blister, which was almost unheard of. From the moment we landed in Kathmandu, Nepal's capital, we hit the spiritual ground running visiting holy sites, receiving monk blessings and tasting local cuisine. We met our Sherpa team and sparingly repacked in our custom yellow duffel bags for the donkey's trek ahead. And just like that, an early morning helicopter departure whisked us away into the Himalayan mountains.

Sharing the road with many kindred spirits, it took all of our energy to rally every day for our endless walks on well-worn trails. (You could not get lost or make a wrong turn on those beautiful, well-marked trails. Thanks to another project headed by Johan, refuse and recycling containers are within easy reach along the way and the trails are kept perfectly maintained.) Each hike filled our hearts and souls with new energy, insights, friends and knowledge. Nothing makes you grow as a human more than stepping outside your comfort zone. It's a part of our evolution to walk into uncomfortable situations. And that's the beauty of my trips…to grow and develop.

The extraordinary trail from Lukla over the river and through the woods to Goyko was a very well-executed acclimatizing ascent to the top of the world in seven days. But, arriving into the thriving "big village" of Namche for two nights in between was the highlight of the trek for many of us. Rambling around the Namche Bazar, we bought gifts to bring home and one of the girls took advantage of a hair salon to freshen up—an unexpected perk in the middle of roughing it. On our last morning in Namche we headed towards the dividing point between those going to Everest Base Camp or with us to Goyko at sixteen thousand feet.

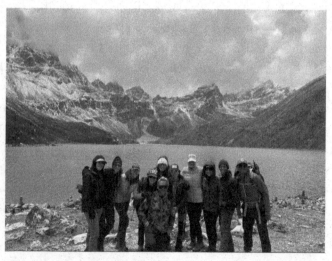

Nine of us eleven trekkers at a crystalline Himalayan lake with our guide Johan Ernst and a Sherpa (far right). The walkie-talkie seen on the Sherpa's backpack was the only means of communication between Johan and the Sherpas in this (refreshingly) no-phone-signal wilderness in the clouds. *(Photo: Author's Archive)*

Altitude is real and my headache was fierce. Staying hydrated and moving slowly while taking it all in was the key to success. We were all in this together and feeling good was high on our radar. This was hard hiking, but there was no rush as we had all day to get from lodge to lodge and we always left early enough to make it before dark. Our undying mantra was *one foot in front of the other*. Johan was patient, kind, motivating, and had answers at every turn. One of the girls got sick the second-to-last night and had to stay back at the lodge, alone. We arranged for a helicopter to pick her up the following morning to meet us. Johan assured her that she needed to stay because she was not strong enough for the next leg of the trail. Altitude sickness can be deadly, and he never took chances. He left one of the Sherpas at the lodge to be nearby and reassure her that all was well.

The Sherpas Johan had hired many times obviously loved him, as did the rest of the locals. Everywhere we went was a Johan love fest. And every night when the conversation got a little dull at dinner because we were all exhausted after hiking seven hours, he would say, "Do you want to hear a story?"

"Yes, Daddy, tell us a story!"

He would tell us adventure tales like the time he walked across Africa. And about his kayak trip through Denmark into Sweden, when at one point he came to some locks that couldn't be crossed. He refused to turn around, telling the waterway constable that nothing is impossible. He found a way by kayaking beneath the locks through the sewer system. One of his stories about helping Nepal rebuild after the ravaging 2015 earthquake ramped up our anticipation for reaching a specific village. We were thrilled to soon visit the Buddhist monastery he helped reconstruct after it had been almost completely destroyed. The monastery is the heart of the community, the social center, and we made a heartfelt connection to that little village sixteen thousand feet up in the sky. Our support of Johan's local initiative made up the philanthropic part of the trip.

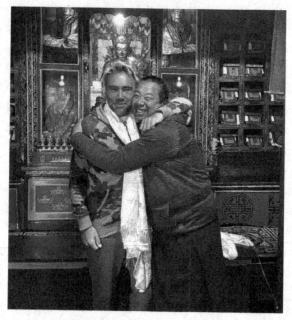

Johan reunited with a monk, one of his many Nepalese friends. *(Photo: Author's Archive)*

Conversations about love and life were as therapeutic as it gets in the awe-inspiring scenery. It rained, sleeted, and snowed, but there's no such thing as bad weather if you are prepared. It was all part of the journey, and we were ready to receive. Three of my superstars made it to Goyko Ri at seventeen thousand five hundred feet on the last morning at sunrise, headlamps and all. Departure day gifted us with the clearest weather of the trip— nice timing, as we were lucky to helicopter around Everest at twenty-nine thousand feet for the view of our lives before heading home.

I feel deeply honored to have experienced this part of the world with this special group of ladies. We felt our strength in numbers and our resilience in spades. This trip of a lifetime will forever live in our souls way after our return to normal life. I loved that we ended up in Dwarika's Himalayan Shangri-La Village Resort for our last stop in paradise together to sit in a salt and crystal cave, enjoy therapeutic singing bowls, chakra therapy, and even see an Ayurvedic medicine doctor.

It was a perfect ending to the rigor of the trek and the beginning of an appreciation of our life going forward. The memories we created and the intentions we set together in the Himalayan mountains formed a bond that will never be broken. Kudos to Johan for taking on his first all-female group, for all his philanthropic work in Nepal and beyond, and for bringing us into his orbit. The stories will keep us entertained for decades or until we meet again.

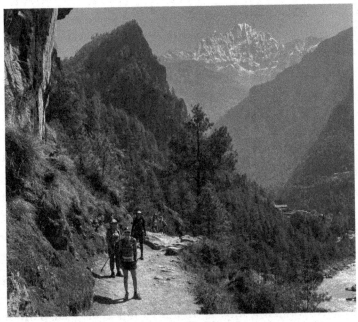

Dry trail, sparkling river below, and the Himalayas all around—
does it get any better than this? *(Photo: Author's Archive)*

A YEAR-END PIVOT

After the Nepal trip I revisited my plans for the STAT trip to Bolivia scheduled for November 2022. The twelve of us were to fly into La Paz, the capital city perched on an elevation of nearly fourteen thousand feet. Dealing with the heights of Nepal, where a couple of the girls experienced altitude sickness, convinced me we wouldn't have enough time to acclimate to this level. Based on my new awareness about high elevations, landing in La Paz would likely mean a huge risk of altitude sickness of one degree or another. Next, I learned that most flights going into Bolivia were cancelled, with the few remaining involving long-wait, complicated connections and arriving at 3:00 a.m.. That meant we would sleep away our first precious day. The third factor in my decision came from my massage therapist, a big adventurous soul who will go anywhere. When I told him about Bolivia, he said, "What? Are you nuts landing twelve girls at fourteen thousand feet? I don't think that's a good idea."

After all those signs aligned, I happened to have a chat with my neighbor who said she just got back from Ojai: "There's such an amazing vortex of energy there—have you ever been?" I did my research and felt the stars lining up to point to California. I asked my Bolivia clients if they were game for the change, and they all said yes. My first choice for accommodations was a winery, but I soon realized it was too small for our group. Then a stunning rental property came up out of the blue and everything started to come together. We made a total Bolivia–Ojai pivot, and everybody was on board, which was the best thing about it.

Ojai, just ninety minutes north of Los Angeles, has the perfect blend of nature and small town charm in the heart of a region renowned for its beauty, spirituality, and ecological harmony. The town's name is derived from the Chumash word for "moon," chosen by the Native American people who settled in the area some five thousand years ago. My STAT ladies added their own vortex of good energy every day in our brief but rewarding stay in a lovely spot overlooking the Topatopa mountains. None of us will forget our first sunset together, when Ojai's famous "pink moment" appeared over the mountains to the north to radiate a luminescent shade of salmon.

Our mornings and early afternoons were spent hiking with our guide, Peter, and his trusty dog, Miley, across routes such as Sisar Canyon Trail with its tall oak canopies, boulder-filled creek, and spectacular view of the Topatopa range. Almost—and maybe just as—memorable was getting around in Dutch's van, a fourteen-seater owned and operated by a local from Amsterdam who decked it out with a karaoke system and plenty of room for dancing beneath the ceiling hand grips and raising a real ruckus. Some of my girls were downright crazy. Good crazy, letting loose crazy. And that's what it's all about, laughter and openness and vulnerability, dancing like nobody's watching. What could be better than a long weekend of blue skies, heart stopping scenery, fearless dance moves, massive amounts of good food and drink, momentous healing, and enormous jolts of feminine energy coming together to seal friendships and create new ones?

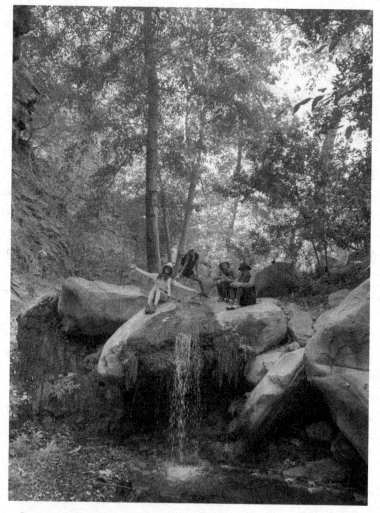

Resting in a canopied waterfall fairyland in Ojai, California. *(Photo: Author's Archive)*

My preparation for the trip included finding local energy workers to offer a variety of healing modalities. I paired up my girls with healers according to their personalities, since I knew several of my travelers well. Fortunately, I found an extraordinary set of healers including Lisa Gotwals, a Native American medicine woman of Lakota descent, Reiki Master, and intuitive with a medical background in nursing. Another practitioner, Nancy Furst, described herself as a spiritual counselor and intuitive who uses drumming, chanting, and other Native American healing practices in her work. We also had opportunities for sessions with husband-and-wife team David, an energy healer, and Tracey, a Reiki Master/teacher. Karina Duffy, a native of Ireland who had trained with Indigenous healers throughout the world, came to us with her vast experience as a psychic medium, shamanic healer, and life coach.

PERSONAL TRANSFORMATIONS

For Stacy in our group, the energy healing and intuitive messages she received from Karina left her physically and mentally refreshed. Karina predicted she would meet a special man through some work they would do together, an inspiring detail because Stacy had always thought it would be ideal to find a mate through common work interests. In their separate sessions with Stacy, both Karina and David mentioned another work-related issue—Stacy needed to hire another assistant. "I have been stalling on it as I have been so busy with work that I have not wanted to stop and take the time to train another person," she told me. "The fact that both healers brought it up was uncanny and a strong message from source." She followed through to start a search for that assistant the following week.

Two of our travelers, Alison and Tracy, came to Ojai with heavy hearts, grieving the recent loss of their mothers. At the beginning of her session with Lisa, Alison hesitated to tell her that fact, but quickly realized she was wasting precious time. During a difficult emotional time, she said, Lisa gave her the gift of clarity:

Lisa is part Native American, and she trained with her elders. She was almost overwhelmed by the amount of chatter she was receiving from them during our session. Her messages to me were a gift, a gift I didn't know I needed. She hit on topics around my son, deceased father, and direction on a new role with charitable giving in our family.

Alison's experience with Lisa was so powerful at that time of grief that she continued to have sessions with her after the trip and also arranged sessions for her family members who live nearby.

Tracy's mother had passed away two months before the trip, and in her healing session with Lisa she was surprised to uncover older grief, still held in her body, that also wanted to be expressed. She described how the session transformed her, lifting away the pain of her "heavy, numb heart":

> Lisa put me at ease, sharing her background as a Lakota Indian, and then she tuned in to her elders and spirits as she talked to me. She picked up on so many things. The grief for sure; however, it was past grief from my high school years, losing an ex-boyfriend with his best friend (my cousin) in a car accident. She even picked up the name—that was a "whoa" moment. He is my angel, always there, she said. She also picked up my grief from my traumatic miscarriage in 2004. In all my grief-stricken moments, I have either grieved or not grieved in the same way. We focused on how there is no one way to grieve. Everyone does it differently. Even the fact of crying or not crying. We discussed my grief as a water fountain—perhaps its gushing, perhaps it's dripping, but collectively, like a glass of water, it's all there.

We talked about my mom holding my hand my whole life…she would still be there. And I could hold my own hand. Lisa also pinpointed areas is my body that held trauma and grief, so I moved onto the massage table and she chanted in her Indian language to ease the places in my body that were holding the grief and trauma in. Once I got off the table and went back to the main house, I immediately felt lighter in my step and demeanor. I had a huge smile on my face and my heart did not feel as heavy. It was an amazing experience and I still feel that in my heart at this moment.

Lesley also experienced remarkable healing with another practitioner, Nancy. At the beginning of the session, Lesley shared three issues that were predominant in her thoughts. She was looking for insight as to where her next place to move outside of Aspen would be (something that weighed heavily on her) and was seeking balance in connecting with her adult boys who were off at college. She also wanted guidance how to continue cleansing the toxic relationship with male energy and men that she had attracted into her life, including her ex-husband.

Nancy then asked Lesley about her prayer life—when she prayed, who did she pray to? God? Spirit? Universe? Lesley said she didn't have a practice of praying, but if she did, it would be to Spirit and the universe. When Nancy asked her why she didn't pray, Lesley didn't have an answer. Nancy spoke about the importance of having a practice of praying that included speaking your prayers out loud, which increases the resonance of what you are asking the universe for. She also relayed that writing was important for Lesley. Writing from a place of being a channel, getting out of her own way and letting the prayers come through her.

I was asked to pick three crystals out of a basket; we did a sage cleansing ceremony; and she also read my cards. Through her interpretation of the crystals and the cards I chose, Nancy was able to give me insight about my questions. She repeatedly told me that I am extremely spiritually connected but I do not realize it because I'm not opening myself up to listen. One of the crystals I picked was shaped like a pencil, which made her chuckle because she repeatedly sensed that I was supposed to be writing. I drew the card of White Buffalo Calf Woman three times. I had never heard of her, but she is the most spiritually impactful Native American woman. Nancy said when something is repeated in a session, such as this, you must listen.

Next, Nancy told her that she was not meant to leave Aspen yet. There was more work for her to do there. She should put that to rest for now and she would know when it was time:

She wanted me to hear that my presence permeates in that town much like the roots of the Aspen trees that are one connected system that permeate the land there. What I had lost was allowing Mother Earth to support me while connecting with spirit. I need to create a practice where I get out of the way, open, listen, and pray. Where I ask for what I want, for help and guidance, and listen.

By the end of the session, they had run out of time for Nancy to address Lesley's last intention about dealing with the toxic male energy she had experienced in her life. "Funny enough," Lesley said, "we both knew I had moved through this, and the question was an old one that I didn't need to ask anymore." She left the session feeling incredibly light and joyful.

When Lesley returned from Ojai, she had a session with her therapist and told him about her experience. As they talked, the idea of moving back into the master bedroom in her house came up. She had not slept there since she and her husband split up years ago. As she spoke about this, an intense, palpable warmth filled her heart, tears came to her eyes, and she knew it was time. She was free.

Lesley now has a daily prayer practice that starts with lighting a candle and feeling herself become grounded into Mother Earth. She asks to open up to spirit, writes out her prayers and reads them out loud. "Then I listen," she said. "I close each session by writing a heart underneath my words. I am finding my way back to the home in my heart."

Each of us was refreshed with new insights from our individual healing sessions, which were topped off each day by long, enchanting sound baths. On our first evening, sound/meditation/breathwork healer Kelly Jean Anderson arrived with her collection of white crystal singing bowls and placed them in a semicircle on the wooden floor. Sitting in the center, she used her mallets to gently strike and rub the rims of the bowls, each one sending out its own rich, luminous pitch. At one point she began singing with her clear, soothing voice, adding to the trancelike vibe in the room. The relaxing sounds pulled us into an introspective and meditative state that literally set the tone for the retreat. We weren't surprised to learn that Kelly with the beautiful voice was a singer-songwriter as well as a healer.

Ava, the yoga/meditation/sound healing teacher and medical technician who performed the singing bowl meditation during our last ceremony of the trip, took a very different approach than

Kelly. Ava wanted to take us out beyond our bodies instead of inward. Showing up with this style of the meditation on the last night was a coincidence in that we were ripe for a more outward experience. We'd been together for the long weekend and already brought our intentions to the surface with our talking sticks and ceremonial sharing. Ava closing out the retreat with that sound bath on Sunday was perfection because she was more of an extrovert. Her energy echoed how we felt, ready to bring our refreshed, inspired intentions and energy out into our lives. But she wasn't done with us yet.

After the singing bowls that night, Ava handed out headphones and invited us to try a newfangled technique called *hypnagogic light sensory meditation*. We trusted her completely, especially after she explained that the hypnagogic (the state between wakefulness and sleep) part wasn't induced by the "medicine" that sometimes shows up in healing retreats. (We never used hallucinogenic substances on my STAT trips—we never needed to. We got plenty trippy on our own.) This light sensory meditation, Ava said, stimulated the brain to release its own DMT, nature's psychedelic. She told us that the technique's ability to ramp up melatonin production, help creativity, and foster deep meditation was making it increasingly popular. Different types of light therapy were even being used to treat trauma, post-traumatic stress disorder, and other conditions. With that, several of us were eager to give it a try.

Ava set up a flat, round light atop a tripod-like contraction and aimed it at my face. I slipped on my headphones, and as soon as she asked me to close my eyes my inner vision was bathed in a brilliant kaleidoscope of lights. The multicolored vision streamed and danced, blissing me out for about three minutes until the music faded and Ava quietly told me to open my eyes. I was amazed when she told me the light source she used only emitted white light. The endless colors I saw were entirely produced by my brain, and I felt as if they'd flown me deep into my psyche to do a cleansing throughout my body.

This was just a brief introductory session; regular light meditations last for about forty-five minutes to an hour. The colors appeared when the flickering light source stimulated my optic nerve to activate my brain's DMT production, Ava explained, as well as my prefrontal cortex, pineal gland, and other sections of the brain. Hindu traditions claim that the pineal gland is a portal to transcendence and connections to higher energies, which may explain why some who do a longer version of this light meditation describe a spiritual sense of oneness with the universe.

The rejuvenating Ojai trip at the end of 2022 was the start of a new path. I felt as if my personal movement into deeper healing was part of the whole world's redirect after long years of sickness. My trips are mind, body, and soul adventures, and I, and maybe many, many others, are moving into a deeper soul connection that will improve our inner health. We're taking stock of where we are and where we're going, getting rid of all the bad muck in our bodies, trying to come to terms with trauma and grief, and moving forward. These last three years have been very challenging, so it makes sense that we would all welcome stepping onto a new, deeply healing path.

It also made sense that the twelve-woman Ojai trip took me full circle as I finished writing this book. Twelve of us had embarked on the Sedona trip all those years ago when my fledgling idea for the business took flight. As the large circle of this story, filled with small circles of gatherings around the fire in unforgettable places, comes to a close, it feels like coming home. A wondrous circle is complete.

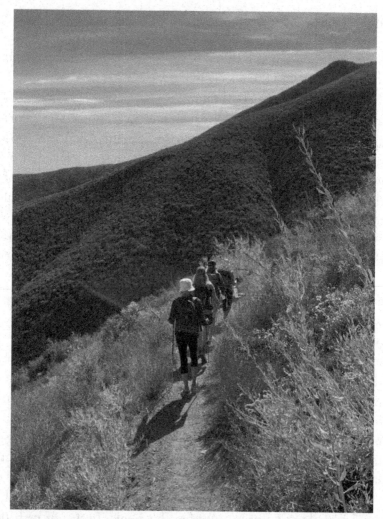

Hitting the trail to round out 2022 in the rugged beauty of Ojai. *(Photo: Author's Archive)*

STARTING YOUR OWN ADVENTURE TRAVEL CIRCLE

I believe travelling any nature-filled path with friends is a powerful way to move into a happier, healthier life. When it comes to some parts of life becoming "permanently different" in the almost-post-COVID era, I hope this book has inspired you—both women and men—to consider making a nature-focused trip with a group of friends. Better yet, think about planning regular trips, once or twice a year, or once a season. You don't need to fly across the country or to a foreign land to benefit from traveling with a small group of friends. The options are endless, from a nearby campground to one of the national parks you've always wanted to visit. The size of your group is also wide open, but bringing together a group of at least three will guarantee opportunities for good conversation and encouraging each other to leave your comfort zones to bike, hike, or canoe, maybe for the first time.

The length of your trips is also up to you—maybe what works best right now is a weekend, or a long weekend, and later on you could do five days or an entire week. These variables are all up for grabs. Researching the possibilities is easy these days—back when I started, there was no internet. I had to physically go to a place to check it out, meet the guides, and feel the energy before deciding to take a group. Today you can do everything online, from searching for ideas to poring through photos and reading detailed feedback from people who've already explored a place. You can also go online to read travel magazines and travel sections in the newspaper in your search for the ideal location. I can only think of one downside to the internet's all-knowing, self-booking convenience: travel agents are no longer necessary.

When you're ready to strike out on your first journey, here are some tips gleaned from my many years on the trail:

1. Choose a place in nature that offers outdoor activities. Even simple walking trails are enough to connect you to the fresh air and nature your body, mind, and spirit crave.

"When we walk away quietly in any direction," naturalist John Muir wrote, "the winds will blow their own freshness into you, and the storms their energy, while cares will drop off like autumn leaves."[6]

2. If you're traveling in another country, look for authentic places to lay your head that are in balance with the place you're visiting rather than lodgings set apart from the local scene. In places like Cambodia or Vietnam, for example, you would miss out on a lot of the rich and colorful culture by staying in a secluded resort.

3. Don't overplan or overschedule. Leave room for spontaneity and the unexpected, because that's when the magic happens.

4. Be thoughtful about whom you invite. You love your friends for who they are, but remember my experience early in STAT when the group vibe in Santa Fe didn't cut it, thanks to some less-than-adaptable attitudes. No one's perfect, but you know who among your friends would probably have a hard time leaving their comfort zone, even for a weekend. Getting along on our own turf is one thing, but it's another thing to travel with someone. You have to be flexible. Things change, the weather turns nasty, plans go haywire. Travel is unpredictable. Choose your travel companions wisely—and if you want to test your friendship or your marriage, take it on the road!

5. Give something back to the community you visit. Do some research before the trip to find out what's needed: donations to the nature park or campsite where you've

---

6   John Muir, "The Yellowstone National Park," *The Atlantic Monthly*, vol. LXXXI, number 486 (April 1898), pp. 515–516.

scheduled your trip, volunteer cleanup duty or other needed help at that park or campground, boxes of items for the closest town's food shelves, or new books for the local library (find out what they'd like). If you have the means to purchase some items, you can look into the needs of a community theater or arts center, animal shelter, school, nursing home, or other facility. My trips have taught me that gifting something to the place you visit is an expression of gratitude that nourishes connection and makes a trip more meaningful.

Setting out as a group of curious and open adventurers, friends can also deepen their connections by including simple rituals on each trip. You can inspire some introspection and conversation by:

- Reading aloud from a book of affirmations, spiritual guidance, poetry, or meditative quotes every morning or evening.
- At dinner, saying three things you are grateful for.
- Agreeing beforehand to bring along an item that represents something important you are dealing with and want to transform, or something you want to add to your life or throw away, and sharing that issue around the campfire or other gathering space one evening.

Each of these rituals opens the door for genuine connection as a tribe of kindred spirits.

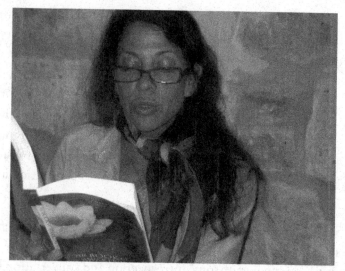

Reading to the group at breakfast on our trip to Croatia. *(Photo: Judy B. Nussenblatt)*

After absorbing yourselves in the wild by day, you can retreat to an evening of tales about the wonders of sunlight streaming to the forest floor and sore feet healed in a cold stream. You can pass around your phones' photos of mysterious rotting logs and neon green dragonflies. And you can make the effort to carve out time for sincere talk that can build a new level of trust, empathy, appreciation, and respect among you.

Dear adventurous spirits, I am 99.9 percent certain you will surprise each other on your close-knit travels. You will feel blessed by the chance to talk with open hearts under the stars. You may find yourselves wondering, "When was the last time we did this—sat together in nature to talk about the things that matter—maybe summer camp? Ever?"

I also believe you'll feel grateful for every minute together. And ask yourselves why you waited so long.

It is an honor to have shared my treks with you through my memories, slices of wisdom gathered on the journey, and voices of some of my happy-traveler friends. Together we wish you Godspeed wherever you trek, both on earthly terrain and in the landscape of the heart.

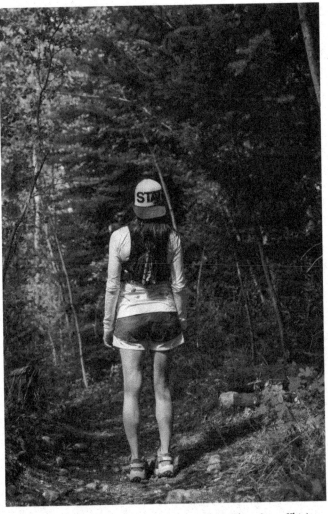

Ready for my morning hike. Where are you off to? *(Photo: Simon Klein)*

ଚଞ

FOR REFLECTION

1. What "pearls" did COVID bring you? How did you change? What did you learn?

2. Do you see changes in any of your friends, parents, siblings, or children?

3. Looking at the friends who make up your "tribe," as you listed them in the reflection for Chapter 10 (question #3), who would be ideal for an adventure travel trip? How could you divvy up the planning? Where would your group go first?

4. What are you waiting for?

BIBLIOGRAPHY

Adyashanti. *Falling Into Grace: Insights on the End of Suffering.* Sounds True, 2011.

Aerogramme Writers' Studio. "Inspirational Writing Advice from Charlie Kaufman,", June 12, 2019. https://www.aero grammestudio.com/2019/06/12/inspirational-writing-advice-from-charlie-kaufman-video/

Airlines for America. "Emerging From the Pandemic, Updated March 17, 2022." https://www.airlines.org/dataset/impact-of-covid19-data-updates/

———. "Impact of COVID-19: Data Updates, March 16, 2022." https://www.airlines.org/dataset/impact-of-covid19-data-updates/

Barron, Susan J. "Depicting the Invisible," Susanjbarron.com, 2021, https://www.susanjbarron.com/documentary.html

Beattie, Melody. *The Language of Letting Go.* Hazelden, 2009.

Beck, Martha. *The Way of Integrity: Finding the Path to Your True Self,* Penguin, 2021.

Brach, Tara. "Resources—RAIN," https://www.tarabrach.com/rain/

———. "Tara Brach on Realizing Your Deepest Intention," YouTube, January 19, 2019. https://www.youtube.com/watch?v=vQHvUVZNIR4&ab_channel=TaraBrach

———. *Radical Acceptance: Embracing Your Life With the Heart of a Buddha.* Random House, 2004.

Brown, Brené. *Daring Greatly*. Avery, 2012.

_____. "Why Experiencing Joy and Pain in a Group Is So Powerful." *Greater Good Magazine*, January 9, 2019. https://greatergood.berkeley.edu/article/item/why_experiencing _joy_and_pain_in_a_group_is_so_powerful

Buettner, Dan. *The Blue Zones Challenge*. National Geographic, 2021.

Centre Yoga. "Nina Reis." https://www.jpcentreyoga.com/nina-reis.

Chopra, Deepak. *The Spontaneous Fulfillment of Desire*. Rodale, 2003.

Clasby, Nancy Torgove. *The Reluctant Mystic: Autobiography of an Awakening*, Small Batch Books, 2016.

Dean, Lydia. *Jumping the Picket Fence: A Woman's Search for Meaning*. Lydia Dean, 2015.

Dispenza, Joe. *Breaking the Habit of Being Yourself*, Hay House, 2012.

Dorfman, H. A. *Coaching the Mental Game*, Lyons Press, 2017.

Edgeworth, Maria. *Ormond: A Tale*. Macmillan, 1895.

Egan, Kerry. *On Living*. Penguin, 2016.

Einstein, Albert and William Hermanns, *Einstein and the Poet: In Search of the Cosmic Man*. Branden Books, 1983.

Estés, Clarissa Pinkola. *Women Who Run With the Wolves*, Ballantine, 1995.

Galvin, Abbie. "The Studio," http://www.thestudio.yoga/ abbie-galvin

_____. *Katonah Yoga Home Practice*, The Studio, 2018.

Harris, Sam. *Waking Up: A Guide to Spirituality Without Religion*, Simon & Schuster, 2014.

Hermanns, William. *Einstein and the Poet: In Search of the Cosmic Man*, Branden Books, 2011.

Hill II, Robert M. and Edward F. Fischer, "An Ethnohistorical Approach to Kaqchikel Maya Ethnopsychology," *Ancient Mesoamerica*, vol. 10 (1999).

Hobson, Nick. "The Emerging Science of Ritual: A New Look on an Ancient Behavior." *Thrive Global*, December 7, 2017. https://thriveglobal.com/stories/the-emerging-science-of-ritual-a-new-look-on-an-ancient-behavior/

Isaacson, Walter. *Steve Jobs*. Simon & Schuster, 2013.

Jefferson, Thomas. *Notes on Religion* (1776), published in *The Writings of Thomas Jefferson: 1816–1826* (1899), edited by Paul Leicester Ford, v. 2.

Jobs, Steve. "You've Got to Find What You Love," June 14, 2005, https://news.stanford.edu/news/2005/june15/jobs-061505.html

Jones, Serene. "After the Fast," September 18, 2021, https://pasyn.org/sermon/after-fast Serene Jones, *Call It Grace: Finding Meaning in a Fractured World*. Viking, 2019.

Jørgensen, Sven Erik et al. *Flourishing Within Limits to Growth: Following Nature's Way*. Taylor & Francis, 2015.

Jung, Carl G. In *Carl Jung Depth Psychology*, May 7, 2020, https://carljungdepthpsychologysite.blog/2020/05/07/carl-jung-on-intuition-and-intuitives-anthology/#.YLmtFC1h0iM

Kluger, Jeffrey and Allison Singer, "'A Year Full of Emotions.' What Kids Learned from the COVID-19 Pandemic," *Time*, June 12, 2021, https://time.com/6071300/kids-pandemic/

Koshy, G. J., K. A. April, and B. Dharani, B. (2020). Intuition and Decision-Making: Business and Sports Leaders. *Effective Executive, 23*(2), 31-65. https://www-proquest-com.ezproxy. mnsu.edu/scholarly-journals/intuition-decision-making-business-sports-leaders/docview/2446289840/se-2?accountid=12259

Kumar, Amit Deep. *Soul Cuppa: The Cup of Soul*, Notion Press, 2017.

Lamott, Anne. *Hallelujah Anyway*, Riverhead, 2017.

Lieberman, Daniel E. et al.. "Running in Tarahumara (Rarámuri) Culture, *Current Anthropology*, Vol. 61/3, June 2020, https://www.journals.uchicago.edu/doi/10.1086/708810

Liebowitz, Jay. "Intuition-based Decision-making: The Other Side of Analytics." *Analytics*, March 2, 2015. https://pubsonline. informs.org/do/10.1287/LYTX.2015.02.02/full/

Linn, Denise. *Kindling the Native Spirit: Sacred Practices for Everyday Life*. Hay House, 2015.

Martino et al., "The Connection Prescription," *Analytic Review*, 2015. https://www.ncbi.nlm.nih.gov/pmc/articles/PMC6125010/

McTaggart, Lynne. *The Power of Eight*. Simon & Schuster, 2018.

Merculieff, Ilarion. "Arctic Traditional Knowledge and Wisdom: Changes in the North American Arctic," Arctic Council SAO Plenary Meeting, March 2017. https://kylewhyte.cal.msu.edu/wp-content/uploads/sites/12/2020/08/Arctic-Council-Report.pdf

Muir, John. "The Yellowstone National Park," *The Atlantic Monthly*, vol. LXXXI, number 486 (April 1898).

Newport, Cal. "What Steve Jobs Meant When He Said 'Follow Your Heart,'" April 5, 2015, https://calnewport.com/what-steve-jobs-meant-when-he-saidfollow-your-heart/

Noodin, Margaret. "A Joyful Life," in Heid E. Erdrich, Ed., *New Poets of Native Nations*, Graywolf Press, 2018.

Oliver, Mary. "At the River Clarion," in *Devotions: The Selected Poems of Mary Oliver*. Penguin, 2017.

Prager, Dennis. "Growing Up to Be Good Is More Important Than Career," *The Daily Signal*, October 1, 2019, https://www.dailysignal.com/2019/10/01/growing-up-to-be-good-is-more-important-than-career/

Rinpoche, Phakchok. "Dealing with Your Jealous and Competitive Mind," Tricycle, August 17, 2016, https://tricycle.org/article/dealing-with-your-jealousand-competitive-mind/

Rowland, Deborah. *Still Moving: How to Lead Mindful Change*, Wiley, 2017.

Rushkoff, Douglas. *Team Human*, Norton, 2019.

Seppälä, Emma. "Social Connection Boosts Health, Even When You're Isolated," *Psychology Today*, March 23, 2020.

Sondhi, N. K. *Small Things Matter Most*. General Press, 2019.

Spencer, Stephan. "Unlock the Secrets of Your Soul with Eliyahu Jian," *Get Yourself Optimized* [podcast], February 22, 2018. https://www.getyourselfoptimized.com/unlock-secrets-soul-eliyahu-jian/

St. James, Aleta. *Life Shift: Let Go and Live Your Dream.* Simon & Schuster, 2005.

Suttie, Jill and Jason Marsh. "5 Ways Giving Is Good for You," Greater Good: Berkeley, December 13, 2010, https://greatergood. berkeley.edu/article/item/5_ways_giving_is_good_for_you

Tippett, Krista. "Brené Brown: Strong Back, Soft Front, Wild Heart." On Being with Krista Tippet, January 2, 2020.

Tolle, Eckhart. *The Power of Now: A Guide to Spiritual Enlightenment*, Namaste Publishing, 2004.

U.S. Travel Association, "Monthly Travel Data Report, March 3, 2022. https://www.ustravel.org/research/monthly-travel-data-report

Vanzant, Iyanla. Twitter, September 3, 2012, @lyanlavanzant.

_____. *Until Today! Daily Devotions for Spiritual Growth and Peace of Mind.* Atria/Simon & Schuster, 2000.

Weave: The Social Fabric Project. "Why I Started Weave, An Interview with David Brooks." The Aspen Institute, 2020, https://weareweavers.org/weavers/why-i-started-weave-an-interview-with-david-brooks/

Wright, Josh. "Letting Go." February 12, 2014, https://www.joshwrightpiano.com/blog/letting-go

"'You've got to find what you love,' Jobs says," *Stanford News*, June 14, 2005. https://news.stanford.edu/2005/06/14/jobs-061505/

"Whitewashed Hope," *Cultural Survival*, November 24, 2020. https://www.culturalsurvival.org/news/whitewashed-hope-message-10-indigenous-leaders-and-organizations

ACKNOWLEDGMENTS

So many people helped me with this book in so many ways. Thank you to Antonia Felix, my writer, my editor, my sounding board and now my dear friend for making my words sing on every page of this book. You are an incredible talent and I'm forever grateful that you took me on. And to my agent Paul Fedorko for the introduction to Antonia and for trusting the project wasn't "just another female story."

To my beloved STAT community, thank you for sharing your personal stories with me and letting me share them with my readers. It's an honor to have taken you out of your comfort zones with your permission. A special thanks to Judy Nussenblatt, my intrepid traveler who shared some of her stunning STAT trip photography for this book. And to Susan J. Barron for her professional photography and showcasing of our talking sticks.

I'm so grateful to all my mentors along the way that have helped me create a meaningful life. They inspire me to be better in everything I do.

Thank you to everyone at Post Hill Press for always bringing their best to this project from start to finish—your expertise and attention to detail have made all the difference.

And thank you to my husband, Paul, and my boys, Spencer and Sheldon. I wrote this book for you. All those trips I made without you were indeed "business trips" that contributed to my personal well-being and purpose in order to be the best wife and mother.

ABOUT THE AUTHOR

ERIN LEIDER-PARISER BEGAN HER wellness career training as a fitness instructor in Los Angeles and working as a personal trainer to the stars in New York City. She earned a master's degree in exercise physiology at Columbia University and a few years later launched Sports Travel Adventure Therapy (STAT). For nearly thirty years, Erin has led STAT trips on all seven continents, facilitating life-changing experiences for hundreds of women, as well as additional trips for couples, friends, and family. She and her husband have two sons and live in New York City and Aspen.

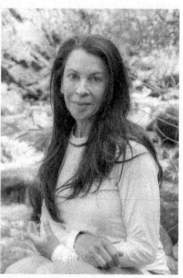

Photo credit: Simon Klein